LIFE'S LITTLE TOOLBOX

First published in 2003

Allen & Unwin
83 Alexander Street
Crows Nest NSW 2065
Australia
Phone: (61 2) 8425 0100
Fax: (61 2) 9906 2218
Email: info@allenandunwin.com
Web: www.allenandunwin.com

National Library of Australia
Cataloguing-in-Publication entry:

Vesk, Nils.
   Life's little toolbox.

   Bibliography.
   ISBN 1 74114 250 4.

   1. Conduct of life. 2. Self-actualisation (Psychology).
   3. Success - Psychological aspects. I. Title.

158.1

Back cover photo by Paul O'Hanlon
Text Design by Louise Davis, Mathematics
Set in 10/12 pt FFScala by Bookhouse, Sydney
Printed by McPherson's Printing Group

10 9 8 7 6 5 4 3 2 1

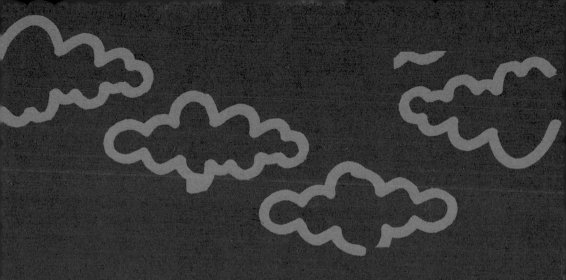

LIFE'S LITTLE TOOLBOX

QUICK TIPS FOR A HEALTHIER, HAPPIER YOU!

NILS VESK

CONTENTS

How to use this book   vi
Introduction   vii
The tool finder   ix

Part I   The mind   1
            1. Mental health   2
            2. Relaxation   15
            3. Meditation   26

Part II   The body   39
            4. Nutrition   40
            5. Fitness fun   61
            6. Yoga   78
            7. Massage   116

Part III   The spirit   127
            8. The real you   128
            9. Choices   141
            10. Expression   152

Conclusion   164
Recommended reading and resources   166
Acknowledgments   171

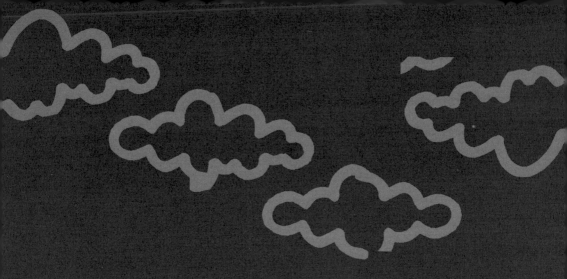

HOW TO USE THIS BOOK

This book is full of tools to help you to live your life to the full. You can read it from beginning to end, or flick through the tool finder to find the right tool to help you with your specific problem.

Throughout each chapter, you will find practical, fun exercises designed to give you the tools for dealing with life's dilemmas.

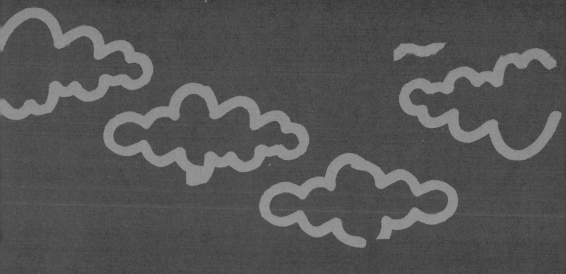

INTRODUCTION

Want to feel better? Who doesn't!?! But how many of us make time to feel better? This book gives you shortcuts, a toolbox of shortcuts, so you don't have to read encyclopaedias on each topic covered to find ways of dealing with life's dilemmas.

I live an amazing life full of all kinds of adventures, doing what I love to do. There was a point in my life when everything started to happen for all the right reasons. Since then, everything has been about doing what I love. This book is one of those loves, helping people to transform their own lives so they can live one that is exceptional.

How do you live an exceptional life, and where do you start?

Life for me is all-encompassing. I believe everything we do, every moment we have, is an opportunity. If we can find out what makes us feel content and happy, we can also empower ourselves to do what we really love.

This toolbox is designed to help you take charge of your life and transform yourself to live an exceptional life. You will find out how the body, mind and spirit work together. You will realise how wonderful you already are and how much more you can get out of life.

I have been fortunate to have learnt much from the many facets of my life, spending lots of time and energy in getting to where I am. I always wonder how certain pieces of information go straight to the heart of the matter, telling me exactly what I needed to know at the right time. This book is designed to do just that, to help you when you are stuck, to inspire you when you are feeling low and to let you discover the things that you really love. It is like hitching a ride to living an extraordinary life.

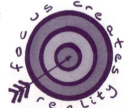

I hope you enjoy this journey . . .

Bon voyage,
Nils

Log on the website www.lifeslittletoolbox.com to find out about workshops and events.

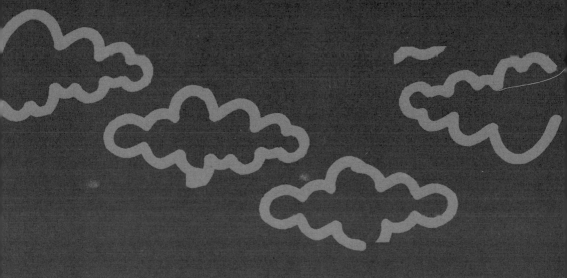

THE TOOL FINDER

HOW TO FIND THE RIGHT TOOLS FOR YOUR COMMON PROBLEMS?

POOR MOTIVATION

DON'T HAVE THE ENERGY TO OPEN YOUR EYELIDS?

Try the winter (kidneys/bladder energy) yoga Chapter 6 p 108. Read Chapter 9 'Basic intuition exercise' p 147.

Mental health try Chapter 1 'Procrastination busting tools' p 10. And 'Communication freeing tools' p 8.

CAN'T CONCENTRATE

COULDN'T THROW A DART AT AN ELEPHANT.

Try the spring (liver/gall bladder energy) yoga Chapter 6 p 92. Try the 'mantra' meditation Chapter 3 p 33. Let off some steam, and do a cardiovascular work-out; see Chapter 5 p 66 for guidance.

CAN'T GET ORGANISED

COULDN'T EVEN ORGANISE A TAKEAWAY PIZZA?

Try the spring (liver and gall bladder energy) yoga Chapter 6 p 92. Read 'Time management tools' Chapter 1 p 12.

BEEN PROCRASTINATING

REALISED IT WAS TIME TO SEE THE DENTIST WHEN YOUR TOOTH FELL OUT!

Mental health try Chapter 1 'Procrastination busting tools' p 10. Try the winter (kidneys/bladder energy) yoga Chapter 6 p 108.

STRESSED OUT

YOU'RE NOT EVEN 30, YET YOU'RE FINDING GREY HAIRS!

Try the winter (kidneys/bladder energy) yoga Chapter 6 p 108. Read Chapter 2 Relaxation p 16. Mental health try Chapter 1 'Time management tools' p 12 and

'Communication freeing tools' p 8. Try the neck and shoulders massage Chapter 7 pp 121 and 118.

CAN'T COPE

YOU LEAVE TWO TROLLEYS OF GROCERIES AT THE SUPERMARKET WORRYING IF YOUR PARTNER IS HAVING AN AFFAIR!
Read Chapter 2 Relaxation p 16. Try the winter (kidneys/bladder energy) yoga Chapter 6 p 108. Neck and shoulders massage Chapter 7 pp 121 and 118. Read Chapter 1 'Communication freeing tools' p 8. See 'Sunrise notes' Chapter 10 p 153.

DEPRESSED

FEELING DOWN AND OUT!
Try the summer (heart energy) yoga Chapter 6 p 96. Read Chapter 10 Expression p 153. Look at 'Communication freeing tools' Chapter 1 p 8. Talk to a counsellor or psychologist.

LONELY

YOU LISTEN TO LOVE SONG DEDICATIONS EVERY NIGHT!
Try the late summer (stomach/spleen energy) yoga Chapter 6 p 100. Look at 'Communication freeing tools' Chapter 1 p 8. Read Chapter 10 Expression p 153.

SCARED

WORRYING TOO MUCH, SCARED OF BEING ROBBED OR MUGGED?
Try the winter (kidneys/bladder energy) yoga Chapter 6 p 108. Read Chapter 8 The real you p 129. Read Chapter 10 Expression p 153.

ANGRY

COULD TEAR OUT THE HEART OF A LION WITH YOUR BARE HANDS!
Try the spring (liver and gall bladder energy) yoga Chapter 6 p 92. Read Chapter 2 Relaxation p 16. Let off some steam, and do a cardio work-out; see Chapter 5 p 66 for guidance. Read Chapter 10 Expression p 153.

FRUSTRATED

BEEN TAKING ONE STEP FORWARDS AND TWO STEPS BACKWARDS!

Try the winter (kidneys/bladder energy) yoga Chapter 6 p 108. Read Chapter 9 'Focus and belief create your reality' p 143.

SAD

JUST WANT TO CRY!

Look at 'Communication freeing tools' p 8. Read Chapter 10 Expression p 153. Do some summer (heart energy) yoga Chapter 6 p 96.

NERVOUS

SPENDING MORE TIME IN THE TOILET THAN ANYWHERE ELSE!

Try the winter (kidneys/bladder energy) yoga Chapter 6 p 108. Try the neck and shoulders massage Chapter 7 pp 121 and 118. Try the meditations in Chapter 3 p 27. Read Chapter 2 Relaxation p 16.

STUPID

NO-ONE WILL LISTEN TO ME, NOT EVEN THE DOG!

Look at 'Communication freeing tools' p 8. Read Chapter 10 Expression p 153. Do some summer (heart energy) yoga Chapter 6 p 96. Let off some steam, and work out; see Chapter 5 for guidance p 62.

STORMY DAY

EVERYTHING THAT CAN GO WRONG HAS GONE WRONG!

Read Chapter 2 Relaxation p 16. Let off some steam, and work out; see Chapter 5 for guidance p 62. Look at 'Communication freeing tools' p 8. Read Chapter 9 'Focus and belief create your reality' p 143.

When things aren't going right with the body

Feel fat

Feeling bigger (a lot bigger) than you want to be!

Do something physical Chapter 5 p 62. Read Chapter 4 Nutrition p 41. Try the autumn (large intestine/lung energy) yoga Chapter 6 p 104. Read Chapter 9 p 142.

Sick

Feeling green and ready to hurl!!

See a doctor! Sorry you probably need to hurl as well.

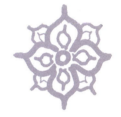

Stiff and sore joints

Feeling like the 'Tin Man' from the Wizard of Oz!

Try the spring (liver/gall bladder energy) yoga and the stretch class in Chapter 6 pp 92 and 84. Try the massages in Chapter 7 p 117.

Aches and pains

Feeling like you've been a pincushion!

Try the spring (liver/gall bladder energy) yoga p 92 in Chapter 6. Try the massages in Chapter 7 p 117.

Sore neck

Feeling like your head's leaning over like the Tower of Pisa!

Try the neck massage in Chapter 7 p 121. Try the winter (kidneys/bladder energy) yoga Chapter 6 p 108.

RSI

BEEN WORKING TOO HARD WITH THE COMPUTER MOUSE!

Try the summer yoga Chapter 6 p 96. Look at Chapter 1 Mental health, in particular 'Stress identification and management tools' p 3 and 'Time management tools' p 12.

FLU

FEELING BAD INSIDE AND OUT!

Try the autumn (large intestine/lung) energy yoga Chapter 6 p 104. See Chapter 4 for guidance on good nutrition, as it affects your feelings, p 41.

COUGHS AND COLDS

ONE MORE COUGH AND YOUR THROAT WILL COLLAPSE!

Try the late summer (stomach/spleen energy) yoga Chapter 6 p 100. Make sure your diet is good; see Chapter 4 for guidance p 41.

LIBIDO

JUST CAN'T GET IT UP OR HE SEEMS TO ENJOY HIMSELF BUT YOU DON'T!

Try the winter (kidneys/bladder energy) yoga Chapter 6 p 108. Eat the right foods; see Chapter 4 for guidance p 41. Look at 'Communication freeing tools' p 8. Read Chapter 10 Expression p 153.

JUNK FOOD ADDICTION

SHOULD YOU HAVE VIP DISCOUNTS AT FAST-FOOD CHAINS BECAUSE YOU EAT THERE SO OFTEN?

Try the late summer (stomach/spleen energy) yoga Chapter 6 p 100. Read Chapter 4 Nutrition p 41.

SWEET ADDICTION

SUGAR BABY!

Try the late summer (stomach/spleen energy) yoga Chapter 6 p 100. Read Chapter 4 Nutrition p 41.

Feeling old day

Especially on certain birthdays!
Try the winter (kidneys/bladder energy) yoga Chapter 6 p 108. Read Chapter 9 Choices p 142. Do something physical Chapter 5 p 62.

Drug addiction

Need a little more to get you going, or to feel real cool!
Try the spring (liver and gall bladder energy) yoga Chapter 6 p 92. Look at 'Communication freeing tools' p 8. Read Chapter 10 Expression p 153. Try a meditation from Chapter 3 p 27.

Sore back

Why does it feel like I have two backs, an upper and lower back?
Do the back warm-up class p 88 and the stretch class p 84 in Chapter 6. Try the massages in Chapter 7 p 117.

When things aren't going well with your spirit

Frustration

Not getting what you want!
Read Chapter 9 Choices p 142. Read Chapter 2 Relaxation p 16. Let off some steam, and do a cardio work-out; see Chapter 5 p 62 for guidance. Read Chapter 10 Expression p 153. Do the spring (liver and gall bladder energy) yoga Chapter 6 p 92.

Feeling greedy

I want this and I want that!
Try the spring (liver/gall bladder energy) yoga Chapter 6 p 92. Read Chapter 8 The real you p 129. Try a meditation in Chapter 3 p 27.

FEELING GUILTY

I COULDN'T REALLY DO THIS, COULD I?

Read Chapter 8 The real you p 129. Try a meditation in Chapter 3 p 27. Read Chapter 9, in particular 'Receiving your creations' p 149.

FEELING UNINSPIRED

IS THERE ANYTHING BETTER THAN PACKING CONDOMS FOR A LIVING?

Read Chapter 8 The real you p 129. Read Chapter 9, in particular 'Focus and belief create your reality' p 143. Try the winter (kidneys/bladder energy) yoga Chapter 6 p 108.

FEELING LAZY

ONE OF THESE DAYS I'LL MOW THE LAWN!

Read Chapter 8 The real you p 129. Try the winter (kidneys/bladder energy) yoga Chapter 6 p 108. Read Chapter 1 'Procrastination busting tools' p 10.

FEELING NEEDY

NO-ONE WANTS TO HELP ME!

Try the late summer (stomach/spleen energy) yoga Chapter 6 p 100. Read Chapter 4 Nutrition p 41. Read Chapter 9, in particular 'Focus and belief create your reality' p 143. Look at Chapter 1 'Communication freeing tools' p 8. Read Chapter 10 Expression p 153.

LOST YOUR JOB DAY

HOW AM I GOING TO PAY THE MORTGAGE NOW!

Let off some steam, and work out, Chapter 5 p 62. Read Chapter 2 Relaxation p 16. Look at Chapter 1 'Communication freeing tools' p 8. Read Chapter 9, in particular 'Focus and belief create your reality' p 143.

EVERYTHING GOES WRONG DAY

LOCKED THE KEYS IN THE CAR, GOT A PARKING FINE!

Read Chapter 2 Relaxation p 16. Read Chapter 9, in particular 'Focus and belief create your reality' p 143. Look at Chapter 1 'Communication freeing tools' p 8. Read Chapter 10 Expression p 153.

BLUE DAY

I JUST FEEL AWFUL TODAY!

Read Chapter 8 The real you p 129. Do the autumn (large intestine/lung energy) yoga Chapter 6 p 104. Read Chapter 4 Nutrition p 41. Read Chapter 2 Relaxation p 16.

BAD HAIR DAY

EVEN IF I SHAVED MY HEAD, IT WOULD STILL BE A BAD HAIR DAY!

Read Chapter 4 Nutrition p 41. Read Chapter 10 Expression p 153. Cancel your appointments and get a massage first, then facial then haircut. Wear your favourite hat, and wear whatever outfit you want.

INDECISIVE AND DIRECTIONLESS

I'LL HAVE A . . . NO I'LL HAVE . . . , I JUST DON'T KNOW WHAT I WANT!

Try the spring (liver and gall bladder energy) yoga Chapter 6 p 92. Read Chapter 8 The real you p 129. Read Chapter 9, in particular 'Focus and belief create your reality' p 143.

HATE MY JOB

I DO THE SAME OLD THING THAT BORES ME TO TEARS!

Read Chapter 8 The real you p 129. Read Chapter 9 Choices p 142. Try the spring (liver and gall bladder energy) yoga Chapter 6 p 92. Look at Chapter 1 'Communication freeing tools' p 8.

UNCREATIVE

I WISH I COULD BE CREATIVE LIKE SHE IS!

Read Chapter 8 The real you p 129. Read Chapter 9 Choices p 142. Read Chapter 10 Expression p 153. Do some summer (heart energy) yoga Chapter 6 p 96.

NON-COMMUNICATIVE

NO-ONE SEEMS TO UNDERSTAND WHAT I FEEL OR WANT!

Look at Chapter 1 'Communication freeing tools' p 8. Read Chapter 10 Expression p 153.

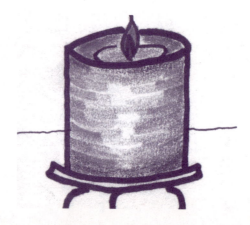

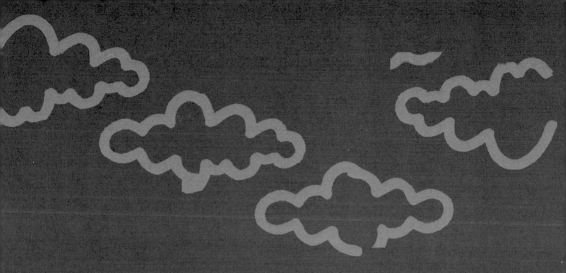

PART I

THE MIND

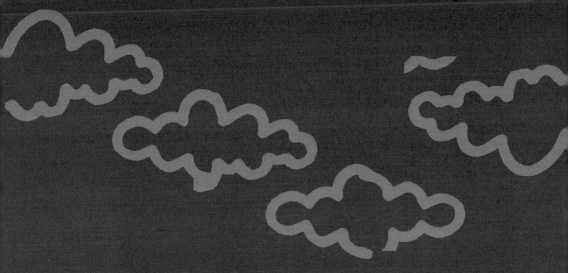

CHAPTER I

MENTAL HEALTH

Most things in life are controlled by the mind—whether we acknowledge that or not is another matter. Someone who is mentally healthy finds that they can communicate and express themselves clearly, are able to handle day-to-day pressures without causing adverse effects on their physical health and are in touch with their emotions.

The following tools will help to ensure you are mentally healthy, your life is in order and you are, consequently, happy.

- Stress identification and management tools
- Communication freeing tools
- Procrastination busting tools
- Time management tools

STRESS IDENTIFICATION AND MANAGEMENT TOOLS

Stress is the most common contributor to poor mental health. It is the force placed on the body by mental or physical hardship. Most people these days suffer stress from everyday situations because they have not learnt how to identify and manage their problems.

You may have heard of the 'flight or fight' response. In simple terms, if someone comes face-to-face with a wild beast, they can choose to fight the beast or run from it. Either way, there would be a release from the physical and nervous tension built by the situation. But, when it is not released, we create within us some nasty side effects. For example, in a workplace conflict, where no physical reaction can take place, the stress is not released. Herein lies the problem.

People show signs of stress but very often they are ignorant of the effects caused by stress. It's not the stress so much that is the problem but how we react to it. Stress can be useful, it can help us get through our deadlines and escape from the beast.

As soon as I am aware of the signs of stress, I can do something about it. I know I get a stiff neck, become short-tempered, eat excessively and my whole body feels stiff and tight. I become more susceptible to illness and usually come down with something. Doing something about it will help to prevent me from getting sick or upsetting people with my foul mood!

Stress affects both our physical and mental health. Side effects can be as subtle as stiff muscles, headaches, poor sleep, poor concentration, anxiety and mood swings. Identifying your stress involves defining your symptoms before they become a real problem: for some people, the first sign of stress is a major one— a heart attack.

How to identify your stress

- Identifying the problem—what is your problem? (This is known as the stressor.)
- Self-talk—are you being positive or negative about the problem?

Identifying your problem

List three major stress sources in your life as in the table below. The more specific you are about them, the more you can do something about them.

Stress Source	Details
1. Book	1. Having to meet deadlines for printing
2. Money	2. Not enough money coming in better work on book
3. Girlfriend	3. Expecting something I cannot give her, not communicating

Well done! You are now aware that stress is affecting you and of what it is that is causing it. Now you need to address the problem itself. Perhaps you have a deadline that is unrealistic. Can you ask for an extension, or for more resources to meet the deadline? You might be worrying about your relationship with a partner. Can you organise some time to communicate with them?

Sometimes we just can't change the situation and in these cases we just need to accept the reality of the problem. Ask yourself, 'What is the best way I can manage this?' Or tell yourself, 'If I cannot change the situation, I will accept the reality', or 'I have done everything I can and there's nothing more I can do.' Ask yourself, 'How can I manage this in the best way possible?'

SELF-TALK TOOLS

When you become stressed, the mind starts to feel the pressure. Before you know it, you are telling yourself you are no good, hopeless or there is no way in the world you can get the job done. This is negative self-talk and it just adds to the tension and stress in your body. When we use positive self-talk, we stop the build-up of stress from within and it helps us to see the light at the end of the tunnel. For example, 'I am doing the best I can, I am working efficiently and effectively', or 'I am getting closer to completing this task'. You need to:

- Recognise when you are stressed/upset.
- Identify the situation which has caused the feeling.
- Identify the unhelpful self-talk that is creating stress.
- Identify unhelpful thinking patterns and beliefs.

Here are some examples of common negative self-talk patterns and positive self-talk to counter the negative.

Extreme thinking: 'If I don't get this contract, I'm a failure.'
Counter: 'I am going to give my best effort to get this contract', or 'I know I can give it my best effort.'

Unrealistic comparisons: 'She always gets so many successful leads—why can't I be like that?'
Counter: 'Am I being biased, comparing myself with people who are better than me?'

It's all my fault: 'I feel completely responsible.'
Counter: 'Am I really the only cause?'

Mind reading: 'She looked at me in a funny way—I must have done something wrong.'
Counter: 'How do I know what other people are thinking unless they tell me or I ask them?'

Catastrophising: 'Whatever can go wrong will go wrong and it will be a disaster.'
Counter: 'Is it really that bad? What's the worst that can happen?'

Fact versus feeling: 'I feel lonely, so I must be unpopular and have no friends.'
Counter: 'I feel this way but what is the reality of the situation?'

Labelling: 'I'm useless.'
Counter: 'What are the facts? One negative should not outweigh the positives', or 'What can I do to change it?'

Once you have identified what negative self-talk you have been using, you need to take steps to help you manage it and therefore manage your stress. Steps to follow include:

- Generate more realistic, helpful self-talk by using the counter talk for each negative self-talk/thinking pattern. Be clear to yourself about what you were thinking or believe about the situation and what you actually know about the situation. Write this down.
- Be aware of the 'shoulds' and 'musts' in your self-talk and change them to 'prefer' or 'like to'. Some of us, myself included, often have a strong set of rules about what we should and should not do in our lives. The problem is our 'shoulds' become inflexible and quite often they are unrealistic to achieve. For example, 'I should be able to find a quick solution to every problem', or 'I should always be there to help my boss, employers, partner, family or friends'. Remember to be flexible, 'I would like to be able to help them when possible'.
- Put it all into perspective. I often get caught thinking that everything that could go wrong has gone wrong. But when I ask questions like 'What is the

worst thing that can happen?', 'If it did happen, what could I do to handle it?', 'Is this situation really as bad as I think it is?' and 'What is the most likely thing that will happen?', I get in touch with reality again, and my stress levels lower rapidly.

Now it's time to move on. Ask yourself, 'Is my self-talk helping me or holding me back?', 'What actions can I take to help me deal with this problem?', 'What lesson can be learnt from this experience?'. This will help you to feel better and move on in everyday situations.

How to release your stress

Because stress affects the body in many different ways, there are a number of different physical response tools available to counter the effects of the stress. These include:

1. Exercise. For a physical release, you don't have to go and run a marathon—check out Chapter 5 for some ideas.
2. Relax. It's not the end of the world—try simple relaxation exercises from Chapter 2.
3. Express yourself and communicate. Nurture your relationships by talking through issues, maintaining a sense of humour, asking for support, talking to yourself as if you are talking to a friend or writing in a journal; see Chapter 10 for effective tools on expression.
4. Look after your body. Eat well and sleep well—try the nutrition ideas in Chapter 4, relaxation exercises in Chapter 2, and massage hints in Chapter 7.
5. Make sure your home and work environments are calm and organised. Try to have a clean and tidy environment. A great way to achieve this is to do small sessions of tidying up during your 'low energy periods' of the day. I always feel a bit flat straight after lunch so I tidy up around me, making sure I have filed documents where they should be, put receipts into my cash book, cleaned my dishes from lunch, put some clothes into the washing machine. You don't need to become compulsive about cleaning, just be clean and organised so that you

know where everything is and other people can find things if required. There is a certain energy that comes from being organised and tidy.

6. Meditate. It will help you on your way—read Chapter 3.
7. Yoga. This is a wonderfully helpful way to release some stress—see Chapter 6.

How do you feel now?
Better? Good.

COMMUNICATION FREEING TOOLS

Communication can save us or ruin us. Effective communication improves our interpersonal skills. It can make us happier, improve our relationships and make the workplace more efficient and productive. With good communication our needs tend to be met, and we are less vulnerable to stress and frustration—it builds our self-esteem.

If we have a problem that needs a second opinion, we need to communicate with another person. We can only keep so much to ourselves—if we continue to hide thoughts and feelings, they can create disaster.

SO HOW DO WE COMMUNICATE?

We speak, we listen, we use our bodies, we use our eyes, we write and even draw. If we aren't getting our message across, we create stress for ourselves, and for others.

How do we receive information?

Think back to your days at school. Some people just loved to listen to the teacher speak, other kids liked to look at pictures all day long, and some only seemed to get the

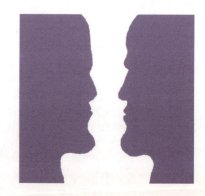

message when a practical exercise or experiment was conducted. These are the three major learning preferences: visual, auditory and kinaesthetic. The population is divided into these three main learning preferences although no-one uses one type exclusively. Visual learners make up about 65 per cent of the population, auditory 30 per cent and kinaesthetic about 5 per cent.

Visual learners prefer written information, pictures, charts and diagrams. They also like to take notes during the learning experience. Auditory learners prefer the voice, to take in what is being said and then write it down later. Kinaesthetic learners prefer to use their hands and bodies. They learn most effectively by copying and practising what is being taught.

If we can find where our preferences lie, we can help establish ways to improve our own understanding of any information being presented to us, and also make sure that the way we communicate to others fulfills the intent we desire. So, whether you are preparing a presentation for a boardroom or a class for school children, whether you want to improve your study techniques or just be understood, making sure that you cover all these learning preferences will ensure your message is understood.

Here are some simple steps to help you to effectively communicate to achieve the impact you intended:

- Speaker—state exactly what you are thinking/understanding, feeling and want; that is, don't keep it in your mind and make the listener guess what is going on.
- Listener—reflect back to the speaker what you think they are saying to make sure the intent was understood if it isn't, ask for clarification.
- Be aware of any filters that the speaker or listener may have which may affect the intent and impact, for example, if they are in a bad mood or are a little depressed.

Assertive communication is the honest expression of what you think, feel and want while being aware of the listener's feelings and welfare. If you can communicate effectively and clearly, you will help to reduce your stress levels.

PROCRASTINATION BUSTING TOOLS

Sometimes, we seem to spend our whole lives running away from doing things that we should be doing. Quite often we avoid doing things that can only be of benefit to us. Procrastination is a serious matter. It can affect our health, relationships and even our livelihood. Here are some examples:

- Avoiding going to the doctor or dentist.
- Avoiding doing your tax return or working on your finances.
- Avoiding talking to your partner about something.
- Avoiding thinking about a client at work because you are too busy.

Whether you are just hiding from what needs to be done, or spending all your energy doing other things, procrastination stops you from really living and enjoying and getting what you want out of life. So let's work on tackling this issue head on.

WHAT DOES BEATING PROCRASTINATION MEAN?

It's similar to diving into the ocean, free from care and concern. You have already done your essential chores, your finances are organised, your business is under control, and you are in good health. Your house is organised and you are on top of everything. You are communicating and expressing yourself. You are living in the moment, not mulling over all the things you should be doing. You are happy!

This is beating procrastination.

Procrastination is like sleeping on a bed with a sharp lump in it. It's uncomfortable but we put up with it nonetheless. Procrastination can be having no money or food in the house for dinner because you didn't get around to organising it. It can mean putting up with a filthy bathroom because you didn't get around to cleaning. Perhaps you have been limping around for weeks with a sore ankle rather than seeing a doctor.

Procrastination may put you in jail for not doing your tax return, or put your livelihood at risk because you have not looked at what your business or finances are doing. Simple chores transform into big ugly issues that still have to be dealt with. You may not sleep well because you are still avoiding what could be some serious or simple issues. These are the bits and pieces that prevent you from getting on with your life and enjoying yourself.

HOW TO TACKLE PROCRASTINATION

- Acknowledge, list and identify what you have been procrastinating about. For example, in terms of health (exercise, illness, wellbeing); mental health (communication and expression, emotions); finance (security planning, savings, superannuation, income); business or work (communication issues); home environment (clean, tidy, organised); social life.
- List what this prevents you from doing in your life, such as getting a new job, new romance, good sleep, more money, improving health and wellbeing, living longer, gaining freedom or happiness.
- List the consequences of your procrastination—is it making you sick, lose money, feel stressed, or affecting your sleep and appearance?
- Acknowledge that you are sabotaging yourself.
- Find a shocking photo of yourself or a monster and deface it even more. Label it 'the saboteur'. This is the part of you that is stopping you from getting what you want from your life.
- Realise that while you can do what you want, your own saboteur will always be hanging around to say you can't. The more you focus on what you really want, the less of an impact this thing will have on your life.

If you feel you're not sure where to start, begin with one simple thing you need to do. Visualise the saboteur mocking you. Now give the saboteur the evil eye. Acknowledge that what you want and what the saboteur wants are two completely

different things. Be aware that you will have developed a pattern that prevents you from getting on with your life. Accept it as part of your saboteur and focus on completing the task.

Do this for everything you procrastinate about and assign a completion date for each task. Focus on what it will feel like to complete the task. Evaluate and list what you have felt while doing the task and then how you feel when it is complete.

Savour the feeling of completion.

TIME MANAGEMENT TOOLS

Managing our time is important. Without time, we cannot work or play. If we can become more effective with time, we will have the time to do what we want.

Just making time to work through this book is a great start.

It is important to acknowledge that we cannot be effective if we work non-stop. If we work for shorter periods with breaks, we will be more productive. By setting a completion date or time, we will be more likely to finish a task.

People have two peaks of concentration in their day. Most people peak around 11 a.m., when their ability to focus and concentrate is best. This concentration plateaus at around 2 p.m., which happens to be after lunch for most people. There is another resurgence, around 6 p.m. These are the average person's peak concentration periods but they may not necessarily be yours. I know my big brother's peak concentration period kicks in around 8 p.m. He swears that this peak is higher than his morning one, and, knowing his early morning mood, I have to agree!

TASK—Record your energy and concentration levels over a three-day period. Simply write down what times you feel very focused, focused, and unfocused. You will soon discover when your peak periods are. With these times in mind, start to plan how you might use your day more effectively. Even though we might have peak concentration times, we still need to meet deadlines and work throughout the day—so how can we make our day more effective? We need to break it down even further to see how long we can effectively keep our attention on the task at hand.

Time management experts have shown that it's hard to keep our concentration on one thing for a long time. We can usually listen to someone doing a presentation for about 15 minutes before our minds wander off, sometimes even to sleep. So how do we get through an eight- or ten-hour day at work? One common solution is to break up the day into hourly blocks.

Additionally we can then break up each hourly block into 45- and 15-minute parts, allocating 45 minutes to the more mentally taxing tasks at hand and 15 minutes to the more mundane tasks. You may already subconsciously have a routine like this and manage your day by fitting easier tasks into your 'slump' times. Experiment and start to see where your day goes, and see if breaking it up improves your efficiency, state of mind and effectiveness.

I learnt a long time ago that beating myself up by working tirelessly on one project without a break stifles creativity and productivity and is exhausting mentally and physically. Being a visual person, I used to do quick thumbnail sketches of what I would be producing, where my time would

be spent, and how I would break up my week and days tackling the projects at hand. It was an easy way of seeing what was still outstanding and what was completed. Maybe you could give it a try.

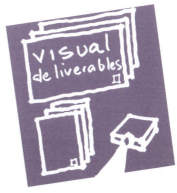

Try to use peak times during the day for complicated tasks and slump times for easy tasks. Set yourself a completion date or time. If you give yourself an hour you might do it in one-and-a-half hours. Yet, if you give yourself no closure time, you might finish it in five hours!

Work backwards from when you have to be finished, organise time, meetings, tasks

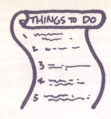

and deliverables. If the outcome is not possible then speak up, get additional resources or reschedule.

All that being said, we still need time to do nothing—to smell the roses, to listen to the wind, to sit and contemplate, to relax and let go. Later in the book I have outlined some ways to help us achieve these great quiet times for ourselves.

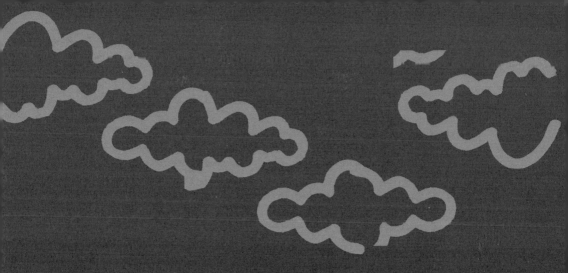

CHAPTER 2

RELAXATION

Relaxation is a state of mind. We are relaxed when we let our mind wander, when we do not have to think, feel and do anything in particular. Most of us know when we are relaxed but we forget to make time for it and appreciate its importance in life. The busier we are, the less time we give ourselves to relax.

Time-out is not just about relaxation. It's about making time to be alone, or to be with someone special, or to be with family or friends. You'd be surprised how such a simple task can give you so much. Time-out has its place even when we are working on lots of issues in our lives. Even if your list of procrastinations is a mile long, you still need to make time for yourself—to watch a sunrise or sunset, to watch the clouds fly overhead and imagine shapes in them.

Relaxation comes easy for some, but others find it difficult to manage. So how do you relax and how much is enough?

People relax differently. For some, reading is relaxing. But if you are reading a thesis that needs summarising for work, this would hardly be considered relaxation! Relaxation can come through going for a walk on the beach or in the local park, riding a bike, or gardening. Whatever it is, don't make it a chore and make time for relaxation in your life.

If you make the time then the rest is easy. Even 15 minutes of relaxation a day is enough. Relaxation is spoiling yourself in a special way. Here are a few simple ways to relax.

MUSIC

Calm music that appeals to your taste is highly recommended. But if headbanging music puts you in a calm state of mind, so be it.

AROMATHERAPY OILS

You can use aromatherapy to create a variety of moods, from relaxing to freshening and invigorating.

Aromatherapy or essential oils are classified as top, middle or base notes. The most effective blends will have an oil from each note. You can create your own blends and here are some good oils to choose from. There are no rules of what you can and can't blend together. Why not give it a go?

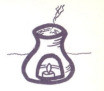

TOP NOTES
Basil—use for memory, concentration, burnout
Bergamot—use for anxiety, depression, burnout, stress and to feel happy
Lemongrass—use for burnout and fear, and to invigorate and create happiness
Neroli—use for anger, depression, stress and to feel happy and calm
Peppermint—use for calming, burnout, concentration

MIDDLE NOTES
Chamomile—use for calming, anger, loneliness, depression, fear
Geranium—use for anxiety, stress, depression and to feel happy and calm
Lavender—use for calming, anxiety, stress, panic
Rosemary—use for burnout, concentration, confidence

BASE NOTES
Cedarwood—use for anxiety, fear and insecurity
Frankincense—use for romantic moods, anxiety, panic
Jasmine—use for depression, stress, burnout
Rose—use for anxiety, depression, stress and to feel happy
Sandalwood—use for anxiety, depression, burnout, stress and to feel happy

HYDROTHERAPY

A bath with Epsom salts or aromatherapy oils, or a spa and sauna, can pamper and revitalise your body and mind.

MASSAGE OR BIG HUG

Getting a massage helps the body and mind to relax.
Sometimes even just a big hug will do!

CANDLELIGHT

We live in an age of harsh fluorescent lights. See how quickly you can create a relaxing atmosphere with candlelight.

CRYSTAL HEALING

Crystals may seem a bit astral to many people, but when you find the right crystal, you really can feel some changes. Even if you are skeptical about the healing powers of crystals, having a small crystal in your pocket can do wonders for you. When you are a little nervous, you can pick up the crystal and play with it in your hand—in this way the crystal can become a substitute for smokers looking to hold a cigarette or it can act like rosary beads.

A FACIAL

You don't always have to go to a beauty therapist for a facial. Treat yourself and you'll feel really good after it and look better too!

EYE PILLOWS

Your eyes get tired so, when they need refreshing, use an eye pillow. It not only helps you to unwind, it also provides the eyes with a gentle rejuvenating massage. If you don't want to buy an eye pillow, you can make one from soft cotton or silk.

Mix 2/3 cup of rice and 10 drops of essential oils—rosemary and chamomile are great ones to use for this. Allow the oil to infuse the rice. Then simply fill a cotton pouch with the rice.

You can store eye pillows in the fridge or freezer and use them on the eyes or the forehead. They not only help you to relax, they can also help to relieve headaches, enable sleep and ease a hangover.

WALK THE DOG

People who keep pets live longer. Giving affection to your pet gives you longevity and it is fun so make the most of it. Pat, play with and cuddle them as often as possible—they'll enjoy it too.

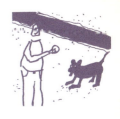

RELAXATION IN THE WORKPLACE

Not only is relaxation in the workplace possible but it is very beneficial to employees. A relaxed, calm and aware person will generally be more productive, efficient and effective at their job. In recognising this, many companies are introducing basic relaxation techniques to the workplace, including aromatherapy, colour therapy, corporate massage, meditation, stress management, fitness, yoga and health and wellbeing courses. Perhaps you should mention this to your boss!

THE LIE DOWN

This can easily be done in the office. Find a place where you can lie down for a few minutes. If you are worried that you might nod off, get an alarm clock or ask someone to check in on you. Close your eyes, have your palms facing up and take a big breath down into your belly. Feel your belly expand and try to push it out a little, then let out a really big sigh. Wait until you need to breathe in again and take another big breath into your belly. Exhale with a big sigh. Then mentally scan your body to see how you feel—are your hands, arms, feet and legs, stomach and so on tense? Relax them one by one. If your mind wanders, bring it back by smiling internally. Refocus and feel your body again. Alternatively, focus on your breath coming in and out or observe your thoughts. This is a mini meditation. If you nod off, you have moved into the siesta stage.

THE SIESTA

The siesta is great when the body is feeling lethargic. The secret to a good siesta is making sure that it's not too long, and waking up in time to go back to work. Unless you live in Spain, it is hard to grab a two-hour lunch break. But we can usually find half an hour or so.

I find siestas work best on an empty stomach. I just nibble on lunch after I have finished the siesta. When I do this, I find that I don't wolf down my food as quickly and I often eat less. Find a park if you can; if not, a quiet place in the office. Lie down and let go. If you can't get to sleep, try a mini meditation and feel the body as in the 'lie down' exercise above. Just don't forget to wake up!

LEGS ON THE WALL

Your work colleagues may find this a little strange, especially if you work in an open-plan office. You're probably going to get teased but it's definitely worth it.

Lie on your back, with your body along the side of a wall. Gently bend your knees, slide your legs up the wall, and shift your upper body so that you are perpendicular to the face of the wall. Place your arms wherever they are comfortable

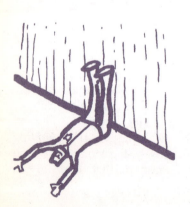

and close your eyes. Feel the blood moving to your head—relax, you won't pass out—and enjoy the rejuvenation and redistribution of blood around the body. What you are doing is reversing the effects of gravity, so stay in this position for a few minutes then slowly take your knees to your chest, twist your body and take your legs down to the ground on your side. Give yourself a few moments to adjust and only when you feel ready, push yourself into a seated position. How do you feel?

THE BREATH

This can be a full meditation, or you can use it in a short amount of time to shave off a couple of degrees of tension. Adjust your posture—you can be sitting or standing—so that it is aligned and comfortable. Take a deep breath and feel your belly expand—push it out a little to exaggerate it—then let the breath go, drawing your belly back towards your spine.

Repeat the breath again, but this time, try to bring the breath higher into your chest. Feel it expanding the back of your chest, the sides and the front. You will soon discover just how large your lung capacity is. When we are stressed, we take very shallow breaths—watch and check this the next time you feel agitated. Keep trying to draw the breath into areas where it has not been for a long time—the top of your lungs, the side of your lungs etc. Just go by the way you feel. Continue for a couple of minutes. How do you feel now?

THE SIGH

Take a big breath into your belly. Feel it expand away from your spine and let out a sigh as you breathe out. Now do it again, but, this time, let out a really big sigh like 'aaaaahgggghhhhhhhhhhhhhhhhhhhhhh ... hh ... !'

Now one more 'aaaaaaggggggggghhhhhhhhhhhhhhhhhhhhhhhhhh!'

A really good one to let go!

HAVE A LAUGH

Are there landmines around your office? Are you starving? Is your leg cut off with a huge gaping wound? I doubt it. Have a laugh, life can be pretty ridiculous, so let's not beat ourselves to death about it. Smile, accept and move on. Do you feel a little bit lighter now?

SMELL THE ROSES

Take a deep breath. What does your place smell like? Hmmm, ever notice how stale airconditioned air does little to make you feel fresh and invigorated? Add some fragrance with essential oils. Here are a few combinations that will help:

- basil for concentration;
- lavender to calm;
- frankincense is an aphrodisiac;
- pine is refreshing.

Make sure that other people in the vicinity are agreeable to the oil you use. If you can't use a burner, you can always cheat and dab a few drops around the place. Try some drops on a thick card or perhaps on your office chair.

TAKE IN A VIEW

Take time to give your eyes a break. If you have a constant range of focus—from close up to far away—your eye muscles and vision won't tend to deteriorate. Try the following.

Look at the tip of your nose, then look at a point a couple of metres away, then refocus on a point a long distance away. Make sure your eyes focus on the point before moving onto another spot. You can alternate between mid, long, short, anyway you like. Also, try to enjoy the view if you have one, or make the time to appreciate something with your eyes during the day. For example, look at a flower and trace its outlines and contours with your eyes. Enjoy the visual feasts around you.

POSTURE

Take a quick snapshot of how you are sitting, standing or moving. Slowly adjust yourself so your body feels aligned. Your head should be level and evenly supported above your shoulders. Look straight in front of you. Your shoulders should be straight not slumped. Your back is relaxed yet upright. Compare this with your usual posture.

Allow your head to lean forward so you are gazing at your lap or desk. Let your shoulders roll forward, how do you feel? Is it easy to breathe? Your posture can really affect how you feel mentally. Try adjusting your posture once more—notice any difference?

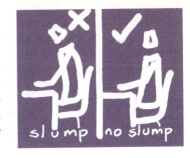

THE SHOULDER, NECK AND HEAD RUB

We may not have the luxury of experiencing corporate in-house massage, but we can still treat ourselves to a very quick massage to release tension. There are some very simple routines in the massage chapter later in the book. With massage you can effectively release tension, making you more relaxed and efficient overall.

THE STRETCH

I love to stretch. I always notice that when I start stretching, people tend to stare, but not long after these same people start to stretch themselves. Why? Because stretching is a natural instinctive activity, but a lot of us have suppressed the desire to stretch. A stretch at work, home or anywhere for that matter is a great way to release tension, prevent injury and feel in touch with your body. Here are some easy stretches to do at the office or home. Also, have a look at Chapter 7 for more specific stretches you can do.

1. The palm tree: While standing or sitting, interlock your fingers and stretch your palms up towards the ceiling or sky. Pull your shoulders back behind your ears. Feel the stretch continue down into your back muscles. Take this even further by lifting out of your hips and looking up towards your hands. Hold the stretch while breathing in and out for a few breaths, then slowly release. How do you feel?

2. The sideways bend: While standing, interlock your fingers and stretch your palms up as before. Keeping your arms extended, slowly take your arms over to the side. Hold the stretch for a few breaths while you look at the back of your hands. Come back to centre and repeat on the other side, breathing freely throughout.

3. The twist: While standing, turn your torso around to the side, trying to look as far round as possible, without moving your hips. Hold for a few breaths then come back to centre and repeat the other way.

4. The forward bend: This is best done while sitting down. Refer to Chapter 7 for specific instructions for the forward bend.

THE TEA OR COFFEE BREAK

If you really want to relax and unwind, tea or coffee is not going to do it for you. Yet you can use the break to give yourself some relief from the pressures of the day. Ask yourself if you really need to have a coffee or tea, perhaps it could just be a drink of water or herbal tea. The most important part is to take the break. If you work non-stop throughout the day, your efficiency wanes, your motivation falls and you feel sluggish.

If you have been sitting down all day, take a brisk walk, throw in a stretch or the legs on the wall exercise above. If you have a snack or drink, take your time consuming these. See it as an opportunity to connect with what you are doing and let go of some of the extra tension in your life. Watch the water as it pours into the glass, listen to the tinkle of the spoon as it stirs, feel the texture of the cup you are holding. Smell the aroma. Feel the warmth or coolness as you swallow the drink.

Put down the cup and consider your posture. Take in a big breath and sigh. Enjoy your break, you deserve it. You will be more productive after a break if you have used the time properly.

The lunch break

This is something you should definitely utilise, not just for food but for a mental rest and time-out as well. Incorporate a siesta or a lie down/meditation, or a walk to the park, into your lunchtime. When I'm really fired up, I'll go for a jog to the pool, do some laps, then walk back to work. This is relaxing for me but may not be for others. Gauge how you are feeling and try to squeeze something into this part of your day.

The car

Driving in the car can be pretty stressful at times but you can make your journey that little bit more calming by using some essential oils/potpourri and listening to your favourite music. Make your car a shrine. Enjoy its company as you would a best friend.

Challenge

Leave work half an hour earlier or on time!
Put some essential oils in the oil burner.
Take the phone off the hook.
Run a bath and include some Epsom salts.
Place some candles around the house, and turn off the lights.
Make sure there will be no disturbances when you finish your bath.
Put on some calming music.
Wear an eye pillow, cucumber slices or a wet flannel cloth over your face.
Let out a big sigh.

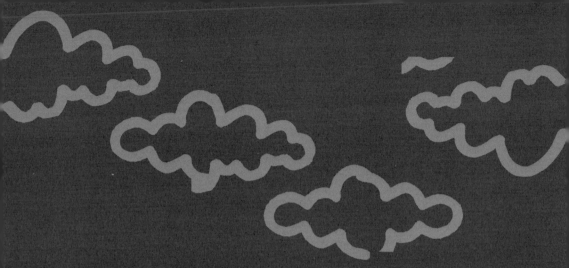

CHAPTER 3

MEDITATION

Do you want to experience peace of mind and enjoy a state of bliss within? These are just two of the reasons why you might decide to meditate. Meditation can also be stimulating for both the mind and soul. Meditators tend to look younger, feel happier and are more content with their lives. They may also find that the skills learnt from meditation improve their personal and professional lives.

Some people meditate to heal illnesses. Others meditate to help them study. Sports people use meditation to achieve a higher level in their field. Artists and creative people meditate to further their inspiration. A corporate executive may meditate to handle stress.

Meditation can also be a means for spiritual enlightenment or religious pursuit. Or it may just help you feel in touch with yourself and your purpose in life. Through meditation, you may start to notice subtle but important changes in your life. You will soon find it easier to sleep. You will require less sleep, and you will start to look younger in the way that people who exercise look younger. Your stress levels will decrease and it may help to lower high blood pressure. Meditation improves memory skills and your ability to accept the different natures of people, and helps you to cope with pressure situations and to generally enjoy life a whole lot more. What else can I add!

What is meditation?

Meditation is the skill of focusing without being distracted. During meditation, your mind becomes so focused on one thing that all the other things around you fade away. Concerns don't bother you; you are aware of them but not troubled by them.

What happens when we meditate?

The brain functions on four brainwave frequencies:

- Alpha—relaxed concentration
- Beta—debate, decision making
- Delta—deep sleep
- Theta—dreaming, heightened creativity

The brain emits these waves at different frequencies, depending on what mode of thinking our minds may be in. For example, when we are engaged in a conversation about politics, our brains will be predominantly emitting beta brainwaves. When we meditate, we are in the alpha-brainwave state. That is, the body is technically asleep but the mind is awake, aware and sensing. This is why we can still get the benefits of sleep while working on the mind.

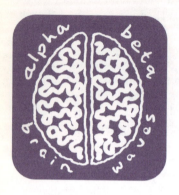

So what? Well, when we sleep we are still conscious of what is going on. Ask yourself, how did you sleep last night? You might say you had a great sleep or that you slept terribly, having vivid dreams. In this way you still recall what was going on because the mind is conscious and slowly ticking over the whole night. But, if you can allow your body to sleep while directing your mind to reach its own 'recovery' state, then you can really recharge your batteries. This is what meditation does.

Don't worry—you will not be out of control, rather you will be aware at all times and can end your meditation at any time you choose.

How to meditate

Meditation can be as simple as listening to the rain and nothing else. Meditation can also be achieved by repeating a word or mantra over and over, creating a wonderful flow of energy through the body.

As a general rule, to meditate you need to get your body into a relaxed and comfortable position and choose a subject and technique on which to focus your attention. This is not necessarily easy so you need to be a little bit gentle on yourself—your harshest critic is you and your biggest obstruction will be your own mind.

One of the hardest things about meditating is dealing with distractions. It's hard to focus on one thing while you are worrying about what to cook for dinner, or when you can hear a dog barking in the background, or if your back aches. You need to be able to maintain focus, no matter how annoying the distractions may be or how pleasurable they are. You need to keep your undivided attention on the task at hand—focus.

Reaching a deep meditative state can be like taking a holiday. But before you go you have to book plane tickets, pack your bags, catch a taxi to the airport, and arrive at the check-in counter on time. Some people never go on holiday as they might not have the courage or focus to do so. Straightaway you discover distractions—other people in the queue, different sounds and sights, or concerns about having packed everything, fed the dog, cancelled the paper etc.

When we first meditate, we have more baggage (thoughts) than any other traveller, because we have gathered so much stuff over time. The seasoned traveller, however, seems to have such a small amount of luggage.

If you keep your focus, you will check in and walk towards the departure lounge, closer to your deep state of meditation. The distractions are still there—a child screams, a custom's dog sniffs some bags and, if you spend too much time focusing on everything else, before you know it you have a new set of luggage and you're back at the check-in counter wondering what happened. However, if you managed to keep focused on the subject or quickly refocus, you will soon make it up to the departure lounge. This can be the start of an inescapable dilemma.

At the top of the escalator, the departure lounge is nice and quiet; you can see the plane. You might be thinking to yourself, 'I like this'. You look around and check out the action, thinking of where that person is going, this and that, then voila! All of a sudden you are back down at the check-in counter wondering what happened again.

When we meditate and things start to feel good, we need to observe any thoughts or feelings that arise then allow them to pass and refocus back on the task at hand—meditating—or we will end up at square one again. By focusing on the task (getting on the plane), we will soon be on board, taking off and flying into a deeper and deeper state. If we drift and lose focus, we need to come back and focus once more without being frustrated.

Your mind will play tricks to prevent you from starting to meditate: 'I've got no time' or 'I can't possibly sit still'. These are usually the most effective times to meditate because that's when you need it most. Take a mental snapshot of yourself before you begin and after you finish and notice the difference—you will be surprised!

WHICH MEDITATION IS BEST FOR ME?

These are five simple meditation exercises:

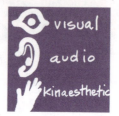

- the breath;
- mantra;
- spotlight;
- watching;
- listening.

The best one for you depends on the type of person you are. What is your learning preference? Are you a visual, audio or kinaesthetic person?

The breath is good for kinaesthetic people, the mantra works for both kinaesthetic and audio types, while watching a candle or flower is great for the visual types.

Some meditations may feel like hard work to you while others seem effortless. Try all of them to find out which meditation interests you the most.

Allow 15 minutes for a meditation. It can be shorter or longer than this—if you are concerned that you will meditate for too long, then use an alarm clock (but not one that is going to make you leap out of your skin).

PREPARATION

For all meditations, find a comfortable position. It may be in a chair that has back and arm support, or on the ground with your legs crossed and a pillow propped under your bottom to keep your back straight. Any position is okay as long as your back is straight. You can do some meditations while lying on your back but be careful as you may well nod off in this position.

Make all the necessary adjustments to your body so that you are comfortable because you should not move during the meditation. Once in position, take a really deep breath and hold it for a moment before letting it out with a really big sigh. Then take another breath, hold it, and let it out with an even bigger sighhhhh!

Now close your eyes and take a mental snapshot of your body. Work your way down from head to toe like a forensic scientist taking photographs. Try not to change anything just yet. Instead, observe the sensations, whatever they may be, as you focus on each part of your body. Become aware of your scalp, forehead, eyes, cheeks and lips then move down your throat and neck, making sure you are aware of all sides of the body part. Become aware of your shoulders, chest, back and down your legs and so on. This is a quick initial examination to become aware of how you feel so you needn't spend a lot of time on it, just a couple of minutes working down through your body.

Once you have scanned your body, draw your attention to your breath. Do not change anything. Just observe your breath as it comes in and out in its own time. Notice how sometimes your breath is shallow and sometimes it is deep. Sometimes there seems to be none at all. Just watch and become more aware of your breath.

Five meditation exercises

These are just a few of the many meditation exercises out there. These simple exercises have been adapted from Eric Harrison's amazing book, *Teach Yourself to Meditate*.

1. The breath

You can meditate using breathing in a number of ways, but a great way to start is by counting your breaths to prevent your mind from going walkabout. After you have done your preparation exercise as above, keep your eyes closed and see if you can give your breath a little bit more space. Can you soften your belly to allow your breath to flow a little bit deeper?

Do not force your breath, just let it flow any way it desires but keep your attention on it. If your attention wanders, just bring it back to your breath, acknowledging that the mind will naturally want to wander.

Count each breath as it comes in and goes out. That is, count 'one' as you breathe in, use the word 'and' as you breathe out, then count 'two' as you breathe in again. Continue counting up to ten, then start counting at one again. If you find your mind wandering off before you get to ten, try counting to five as this will help you to keep your mind focused.

Alternatively, you can count by using the same number for the in and out breath—'one' as you breathe in, then 'one' as you breathe out; 'two' as you breathe in, then 'two' as you breathe out, and so on. Once again, if your mind wanders, just bring it back without getting annoyed and stay with your breath and see what happens.

Continue with this meditation, focusing more intently and becoming more aware of the intricacies of your breath: its rhythm, texture, sound and the sensation of air coming through your nose into your lungs. Focus, but try not to force or will it to happen—just remain aware, relaxed and focused.

When you have finished, keep your eyes closed for a while and sense how your body feels now. Compare the way you feel now to the snapshot you took when you began. Note the difference.

THE BREATH INSTRUCTIONS

- Sit comfortably.
- Note how each part of your body feels.
- Do your preparation breaths: two big breaths and sighs.
- Count your breaths up to ten.
- Continue counting from one.
- If your mind wanders, bring it back and refocus your attention on your breath.
- Compare the way your body feels when you have finished with how it felt when you started.

2. Mantra

A mantra is the use of a word or group of words as the subject on which to meditate. You can use any word/s you like and you can choose to use words with a spiritual or religious context—as long as they make the mantra interesting, rhythmical and musical. The more complex the mantra, the harder the mind has to work to keep focus, and the less likely it is to wander.

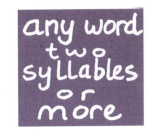

Common mantras:

- Om—a sacred Indian word that relates to the three states of consciousness.
- Hare Krishna—a Hindu god.
- Shalom—a Jewish greeting meaning 'peace be with you'.
- Om manee paymee hung—a Tibetan Buddhist chant.

You can use nearly any word that comes to mind. Once, I used a swear word over and over again after I had a particularly bad day at work. By the end of my meditation there was not a trace of anger or resentment left in me!

Mantra instructions
- Start with the preparation exercise.
- Begin to chant your mantra aloud. As you get deeper into your meditation, you can start to internalise so that in the end there are hardly any word/s spoken aloud but the mantra is still being repeated internally.
- Focus on the texture, rhythm and pronunciation of the word/s. As you focus more intently, the rhythm may start to send a sweeping wave-like sensation through your body. If you like, you can begin to rock forwards and backwards ever so slightly to exaggerate the rhythm of the mantra.
- If your mind begins to wander, bring it back to the mantra. It is easy to say a word but think of something else. You need to maintain your focus on the

words, the sound, the rhythm, the texture, the resonance and the vibration within your mind, skull and body. If you have stopped saying your mantra aloud, perhaps you can start to say it again physically to help you get back on track.

- Immerse yourself in the mantra. You can use the mantra to stimulate your mind by creating a very fast rhythm. If you like, you can start to soften and even stop repeating the mantra aloud—as long as you continue to mentally repeat and focus on the mantra, you will still get the same effect. Experiment to find which method seems to work best for you.
- Slowly end the mantra but remain silent and examine the after-effects—observe what has shifted and how your mind and body feel.

3. SPOTLIGHT

This meditation is an extension of the preparation exercise. It requires you to become aware of your body by focusing on and naming the different parts of the body. This meditation can be led by someone else or you can take yourself through it with just as much success.

SPOTLIGHT INSTRUCTIONS

- Start with the preparation exercise.
- Then focus and mentally identify your right thumb, become aware of it, and any sensations that may arise. Shift your focus to your right index finger and become aware of any sensations. Do not be concerned by how you feel, just observe the sensations as they rise and then pass away to the nothingness from where they came. Shift your focus to your right middle finger, observe the sensations, then move on to your ring finger and little finger in the same manner. Keep your mind focused and simply observe the sensation as it is.
- Become aware of your right palm, focus on it, then shift to your wrist, then your forearm, elbow, upper arm, armpit and shoulder, stopping to observe each sensation before you move on. Become aware of the whole of your right arm.
- After keeping your attention on your right arm for a little while, move your focus to your right big toe. Move through each toe, then to the sole of your right

foot, the arch, the ankle, the calf muscle, the shin, the knee, the thigh and the hip. Become aware of the whole right leg and any sensations that may arise. Stay focused on this leg for a short while.

- Move on to your right buttock, hip and groin. Continue working methodically up the body, intensely focusing as you go. If your mind wanders, bring it back and continue. Move up through the right side of your abdominals, back, chest, neck, throat, face and scalp. Become aware of the whole right side of your body. Rest with this side in focus for a few moments.

- Now shift your focus to your left thumb and then move through the left side of your body in the same way as you did with the right side.

- Once you have worked through the left side of your body, shift your attention to focus simultaneously on both sides of your body. Become aware of both thumbs, and any sensations that may arise. Become aware of both your index fingers and so on. Work up both sides of your body.

- Once you have finished, it is time to start focusing on the inside of your body, using your imagination. Become aware of the inside of your skull, the right side of your brain, and the left side of your brain. Become aware of the inside of your right eyeball, then your left eyeball. Become aware of the inside of your right nostril, then your left nostril, your mouth, your tongue, inside of your top teeth, then bottom teeth, your throat, the inside of your right lung, the inside of your left lung. Shift your focus to the inside of your heart, then the inside of other internal organs, the spleen, pancreas, kidneys, small intestine, large intestine, bladder. Maintain your focus and continue to the inside of all the bones in your body. Be aware of all the cartilage in your body, the inside of the muscles of your body, and your tendons. Shift your focus to inside your arteries, veins and capillaries, inside your red and white blood cells. Become aware of the inside of your spine, and all the nerves in your body.

- Finally, become aware of your breath as it moves in and out in its own time. Notice how sometimes it's shallow and sometimes it's deep. Focus on it. Be with your whole body, just be aware.

- When you feel ready, slowly end the meditation and come back to the space where you started and take note of how you feel.

More meditations

- While walking, pick a point in the distance to where you are headed. I often use a tree or building as my focus point. Slowly start spotlighting on that point. Become aware of your body and how it moves. Focus on and work through your body parts, noticing any changes.
- Try meditating by watching the back of someone's head in a queue or sneak in a meditation at work by staring at the centre of your computer screen.

Even if we only meditate for a few minutes, we will experience a change in how we feel.

4. WATCHING

You can meditate just by watching things—by looking into the flame of a candle, or at flowers, plants, pictures, mandalas or the moon. The basic steps for watching are to focus on the object at hand. Look over its surface, and be aware of the textures, colours and shapes. Do not think about the object, but just watch it as it is.

CANDLE MEDITATION INSTRUCTIONS

- Place a candle, on a safe plate, in front of you at eye level, about 30 centimetres away. Light the candle and turn off the house lights.
- Do the meditation preparation exercise.
- Look at the candle flame and notice how there is a bright light inside the flame (the hottest part of the flame). Focus on the tip of this point of the flame. Allow your eyes to relax.
- If your eyes lose focus, just try to become aware of the rays of light that emit from the candle. Try not to blink excessively. You will find that you can keep

your eyes open without blinking too much, it just takes practice. Keep your eyes on the flame. If any thoughts arise, allow them to, but keep your focus on the flame and then allow the thoughts to pass away.

- When your eyes can't stay open any more, go to the next stage. Allow your eyes to close but keep looking for the light; an 'after image' should appear. The image may not look like the flame, but stick with it. Imagine the flame if you have to. You can mentally name it 'flame', 'flame', 'flame'. This 'after image' may start to change shape, it may become a different colour, just keep focusing.
- If you've lost the 'after image' slowly open your eyes and begin again. Don't be hard on yourself, just focus and let go . . . focus and let go. If you keep focused, you should find yourself in a beautiful space beyond words.
- Record how you felt after you finished compared with when you began.

5. LISTENING

You can meditate just by listening—it could be the sound of wind rustling through leaves or waves crashing onto the beach. If you listen to music, it is better to have music that is complex and without words so you don't think about their meaning.

LISTENING INSTRUCTIONS
- Start with the preparation exercise.
- Listen to the various sounds around you. You don't have to think, just listen and absorb the sounds. Listen to the low notes, high notes, rhythm, texture.
- If your mind wanders, bring it back and refocus on the sound.
- Try to isolate the sounds around you. What qualities do they have? Can you find space between the sounds? Is there something you haven't been hearing?
- Record your feelings at the end of the meditation and compare them with how you felt at the beginning.

Challenge

Try each of the five meditations to find the one that suits you best or alternate between a few or all of them. Then try to meditate for 15 minutes three times per week. You will find that the changes it brings will amaze you.

Keep a diary to record the changes you are experiencing from meditating. For example, you may notice how clear thinking you have become, how well you can handle distractions and how tense you were before you started.

Over time, increase your meditation time—a few minutes longer will make a difference, but, if you can increase the time you spend meditating, you will be able to achieve even more powerful results.

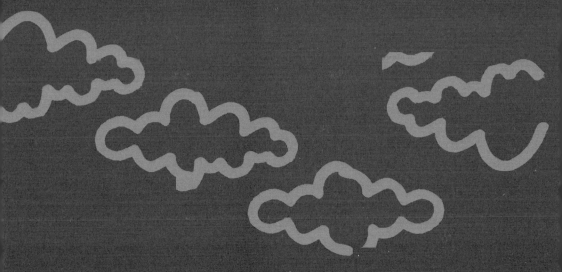

PART II
THE BODY

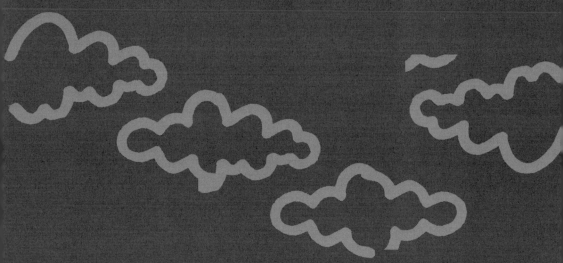

CHAPTER 4

NUTRITION

An island off Japan called Okinawa is home to the world's longest living people. Why do the Okinawans live so long compared with people in other parts of the world? The answer appears to be in the foods they eat, their mental health and physical activity. By studying the Okinawans, much insight can be gained about healthful practices.

Health and vitality are qualities that everyone strives for in our busy time-poor societies. One way for us to live a longer and more fulfilled life is to emulate some of the practices of the longest living humans. When we combine the knowledge of the Okinawans with what we have learnt through many years of research into the effects of nutrition on the body, we can create a way of eating that gives us the energy and longevity that we crave.

This does not mean that we have to adopt an Okinawan diet to live healthily. In this chapter we will shine the light of truth on what food guidelines work for us, so we can apply these to our everyday lives and reap all the benefits on offer from our bountiful food supplies.

THE IMPORTANCE OF NUTRITION

The foods you choose to eat can really affect the quality of your life. Obviously we need to eat and drink to survive, yet we can either 'live to eat' or 'eat to live'. I choose to look at foods and cooking with an end result in mind. I ask myself 'What do I want to get out of this meal? Is it fuel for the body? A supplement of assorted vitamins and minerals to satisfy the body's nutritional requirements? Or is the food to appease my culinary desires and emotional cravings?'

Most of the foods we eat do not help us to keep our bodies in tiptop condition. Many of the medical problems that are widely prevalent in our society are directly related to poor nutrition; for example, diabetes, heart conditions and several cancers could be prevented in most cases by good eating habits.

So what are the essentials? What's good? What's bad? How can we find balance in all the available information?

Because people have different requirements, live in different climates and have different lifestyles, one would be hard pressed to find the perfect solution for all. Yet there are some guidelines that work no matter where you live or what type of person you are. With the help of some experts in nutrition, I have summarised below the most important guidelines to sensible eating habits. I also include the guidelines from what has become known as the 'Okinawa Way'.

At the end of the day, what you eat is up to you, but with awareness and guidance you can steadily improve your eating habits as the foods you lean towards will be a healthier choice.

What is nutrition?

Nutrition is the supply and regulation of essential foods to keep the body balanced or at a maintainable level, known as homeostasis. That is, a healthy intake of food is one that supplies all the vitamins, minerals, protein, carbohydrates and fats which the body needs to maintain optimum health. We can illustrate all our essential requirements by using the example of a fish tank. Inside the fish tank is, of course, water and three big rocks: carbohydrates, proteins and fats. There are also lots of smaller pebbles (vitamins and minerals). This is what we need to maintain optimum health. Let's have a look in detail at the items in the fish tank.

Water

Water is needed for all body processes, including transporting nutrients and oxygen and eliminating waste. Which is why we can't live without water beyond a few days—we can live without food for a much longer period. Water is involved in every part of the body's metabolic processes.

People often misjudge their water requirements. For example, they will feel a sensation of hunger when actually they are thirsty. So thirst is not a good indication of your water requirements because thirst switches off before your fluid levels are fully replaced.

Dehydration leads to tiredness, headaches, cramping, an inability to exercise at high intensity and dizziness. You should aim to drink 1.5–2 litres of water per day and add an extra litre for every hour of exercise, that is, approximately 6–8 cups of water.

CARBOHYDRATES

Carbohydrates are the most effective form of fuel for the body. We use this fuel for all our aerobic-energy activities, such as jogging, swimming and walking. But not all carbohydrates react in the same way within the body. Some are broken down quickly, releasing their smallest component (glucose or sugar) into the bloodstream equally as quickly. Other carbohydrates take longer to digest and therefore enter the bloodstream at a much slower rate. The ranking of food by its effect on the body's blood glucose levels is called the glycaemic index (GI). A lot of foods today are labelled as having a high, medium or low GI.

Carbohydrates that are rapidly broken down are said to have a high GI as they cause a rapid rise in the blood glucose/sugar level, which in turn causes a large surge of insulin to be released from the pancreas and this makes the blood glucose level drop quickly. This fluctuating blood glucose level can give us quick fuel and energy, but it is often short-lived and followed by a slump in energy levels.

Carbohydrates that are broken down more slowly are termed low-GI foods. These foods lead to a sustained, even blood glucose level, which provides a sustained fuel source without the major slump of blood sugar levels. A sustained blood sugar level can reduce the craving for sweet foods, reduce hunger, give you energy for longer and may even be able to balance your mood. If you can reduce high blood sugar

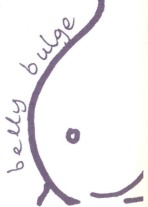

belly bulge

levels, you can also reduce the risk of diabetes, heart disease and some hormone-dependent cancers.

Unfortunately, it is very hard to determine the GI of a food without testing it, but there are several books available that list the GI of foods to help you choose the appropriate carbohydrate sources for your needs.

Basically low-GI foods include fruit, wholegrains, legumes/lentils, dairy products, citric acid (as found in lemons), protein and fat. These foods are often described as wholefoods or wholegrains. Sugar in the form of lollies (candy), highly processed carbohydrates, syrups and table sugar has almost no nutritional value except as a quick energy hit. These foods have a high GI and often when you start eating these foods it is hard to stop. A lot of the food we eat today such as white flour, white (polished) rice, jam and potato chips, is also devoid of natural fibre and other nutrients; these are very low in nutritional value and excessive use should be avoided if possible.

High-GI carbohydrates are not necessarily bad for us, but they are easy to over-consume because their energy is not sustaining. Although the body has some capacity to use more carbohydrates as fuel when we increase our intake, if we eat an excessive amount (more than our body needs) of any food, including carbohydrates, we start to store it as body fat. This would be great if we were about to experience a famine, but in our society it simply means we will have to do more work in the fitness department to burn up the extra energy.

Many people are presently advocating carbohydrate-free diets. Yes, people can lose weight on these diets, but the weight they are losing comes from the loss of water and lean muscle which occurs when the body is not receiving enough energy to maintain its muscle mass. Our fat stores are only slightly affected. A diet that reduces the amount of high-GI foods and contains carbohydrates that are low-GI will be much more effective in promoting weight loss without compromising one's health. Low-GI foods also contain many other useful nutrients.

FIBRE

Fibre is a type of carbohydrate that plays an important part in our dietary intake. It comes from less easily digested plant material found in vegetables, fruits, grains and pulses. Fibre contains nearly no calories, yet leaves us feeling very satisfied—which means we're less likely to gorge on fatty foods and we don't have to expend as much energy to burn it off.

Fibre lowers cholesterol and blood fats while helping to tackle constipation, and it has also been shown to help prevent bowel cancer. A word of warning, though: too much fibre or too great a change in fibre intake and you'll find yourself running to the toilet and listening to the fireworks. If you currently have a very low fibre diet, increase your fibre intake slowly and make sure you meet your water requirements to help prevent unpleasant gut sensations.

We can increase our fibre intake by increasing our intake of wholefoods and reducing our intake of processed foods. Wholefoods include grains, pulses and brown rice, wholegrain products (such as wholegrain or wholemeal breads) and cereals. Eating vegetables and fruits with their skins will also increase your fibre intake. If you don't like these foods, you can always add fibre to your fibreless food—try wheatgerm or bran in your cereal; beans and pulses in your soups, minces or casseroles; fruit in your desserts or breakfast; or choose breads with added fibre.

PROTEINS

Proteins are required by the body for cell repair and to build muscle tissue. Proteins can be found in animal or vegetable foods, and the most important constituents of proteins are the amino acids.

Animal proteins contain all the essential amino acids while vegetable proteins are often low in one or more of these essential compounds. However, by combining different types of vegetable proteins, you can easily obtain the complete complement of amino acids. For example, by combining rice with dahl or peanut butter with bread or corn chapatti with kidney beans, you will provide yourself with the full set of essential amino acids needed by the body. These food combinations don't even have to be eaten in the same meal. As long as you are eating a variety of foods, you will meet your requirements, so you can still be a vegetarian and get the protein you require. The major difference here is that vegetarians have to eat a little more to get the same protein levels as meat eaters.

Good sources of protein include:

- lean beef, lamb, veal, chicken, pork, leg ham;
- fish, shellfish;
- dairy products, such as milk, cheese and yoghurt;
- eggs;
- nuts, tofu, soy products, legumes, lentils and cereals.

Most people eat more protein than their bodies require. A good way to consider how much protein you need is to think back to the hunter-and-gatherer ages. Did they eat meat every day? No, their diets consisted of about one kill a week, so meat would be eaten only about once a week, not every day.

It can be hard to see why too much protein would be bad for you, and how you can have too much, given the convenience of quality meats available at our supermarkets, butchers and delicatessens. However, too much protein puts extra strain on the kidneys, as it is the kidneys that must deal with the breakdown products of protein. A high consumption also increases calcium loss, which in turn increases the risk of osteoporosis and kidney stones. Increased protein, particularly from some animal sources (those that have saturated fat content), can also increase blood cholesterol levels, which may lead to heart disease.

So how much should we have? The average, non-exercising adult requires about 0.8 gram of protein per kilogram of the person each day. So a person that weighs 100 kilograms would require 80 grams of protein per day. An active, exercising adult would require about 1.0 gram of protein per kilogram of body weight. An endurance/strength training athlete would require about 2.0 grams per kilogram, as would a growing teenage athlete. To put this into perspective:

- 45 grams of meat = 8 grams of protein;
- 1 egg = 6 grams of protein;
- 250 millilitres of milk = 8.5 grams of protein.

If you just aren't into weighing your foods, a good way to look at how much you need is by using your hand. A piece of meat about the size of your palm will be a sufficient daily intake of protein. A fistful of rice or pasta will be a sufficient serve of carbohydrates for one day. Obviously, the bigger your hand, the bigger your serving will be; and the more active you are, the more you will need to increase the amount of this simple guideline. I tend to use the palm and fist method for its simplicity.

FATS

Fats are essential to protect the body from injury by cushioning the organs, to carry fat-soluble vitamins and fatty acids, during pregnancy, and as a store for famine times. However, excess fat in the body can be harmful and has been linked to many of the chronic diseases known today, such as diabetes, heart disease, increased blood pressure, sleep apnoea, some cancers and osteoarthritis.

There are three main types of fats:

- polyunsaturated;
- mono-unsaturated; and
- saturated.

Polyunsaturated fats are basically those with lots of double bonds in the chemical composition of the fat, which can simply be thought of as a long chain. They are found in foods such as margarine, canola oil, linseed oil, walnuts, soybeans, green vegetables, fish oils, fish and seafood. Small amounts are found in lean lamb and beef; safflower, sunflower, cottonseed, grains, nuts, seeds, wheatgerm; and soybean, corn and grapeseed oils.

Mono-unsaturated fats have just one double bond in their composition and have been found to be more stable at high temperatures, which may mean that they are less likely to break down and combine with other molecules in the body to create disease. They are found in foods such as olives and olive oil; canola, sunflower and macadamia oils; mono-unsaturated margarine and spreads; avocados, most nuts, very lean red meats, chicken, pork, eggs and fish.

Saturated fats have no double bonds; instead, they have lots and lots of hydrogen ions. They are found in animal products such as dairy foods and fatty meats. The only plant source of saturated fat is coconuts (palm oil is a saturated fat). Saturated fat can contribute to high cholesterol levels in the body, which can lead to heart disease, diabetes and even cancer. Lean animal products such as lean red meat and reduced-fat dairy products do not produce the high cholesterol levels of saturated fats. Polyunsaturated and mono-unsaturated fats are less likely to lead to heart disease and high cholesterol, but they can still add to our belly size.

As a guide, you need about two parts mono-unsaturated, one part poly-unsaturated and half a part of saturated fats in your daily diet. If you use some olive oil, olives, avocados or nuts in cooking, this will take care of the mono-unsaturated fats. The polyunsaturateds can be taken care of by including a few nuts and seeds, fish, or oils such as canola, macadamia and safflower, in your diet.

Fats provide the body with more calories per gram than carbohydrates or protein. This means that the more fat you eat, the harder you have to work to burn it off. Try to limit your fat intake to less than a third of your calorie intake. The more conscious you are of the fat in your diet, the more you can do something about it. When eating, ask yourself, 'Is this a full cream milk? Can I remove the skin from the chicken, or trim the fat off the steak?' and so on.

The good oil on omega-3 fatty acids

Omega-3 acids are a type of polyunsaturated fat and they play an important role in reducing diseases and illnesses associated with the functioning of the brain, the cardiovascular system and the immune system. These fatty acids can help to lower cholesterol levels, keep the arteries clean, and reduce the reactions of an overreactive immune system. People suffering from mental illnesses such as ADD, depression and schizophrenia are likely to have a deficiency of omega-3 acids.

Omega-3 acids are found in fish and fish oils, and nuts and seeds, including flaxseed, linseed, almonds, walnuts, soy nuts (roasted soybeans), and pumpkin and sunflower seeds.

VITAMINS AND MINERALS

Vitamins and minerals are essential as they are involved in breaking down carbohydrates, proteins and fats to obtain energy. They affect our blood quality, nervous system, muscles, hair, teeth, eyes, skin and bones. Each vitamin and mineral has a specific role to play in maintaining the body's equilibrium.

If you enjoy a wide range of carbohydrates, proteins, fruit, vegetables, herbs and spices, you will be able to supply your body with all its vitamin and mineral requirements. However, you may need help if you consume a lot of processed food. The more a food is modified from its original form, the more vitamins and minerals are lost, and the more unwanted additives and preservatives come on board. If you can maintain an adequate intake of wholefoods, you will be getting the most from your food.

A lot of people find it a shock when they initially adjust to foods that are less processed. The taste is different, but it is the true flavour of the food. I find the taste of a fresh mushroom risotto much more satisfying and enjoyable than a dehydrated, preservative-filled pasta dish with an instant sauce.

A healthy diet should not need supplements of vitamins and minerals. If you feel you need extra supplements, be careful as excess amounts of some vitamins can cause serious side effects. Consult a dietician or doctor if you need advice.

NUTRITION—HOW TO PUT IT INTO PRACTICE

Now that we have covered the basics of what nutrition is, we can focus on how to achieve this in our everyday lives. The best way to do this is to look at what the top nutritionists and dieticians have been advocating for the past ten years, including the various published guidelines, ways to reduce your fat intake, responsible alcohol intake, and, of course, eating out.

DIETARY GUIDELINES

Despite the fad diets which continue to rise and fall, the guidelines below are still the basis for sensible healthy eating.

AUSTRALIAN DIETARY GUIDELINES
(published by Commonwealth Department of Health and Community Services and the Health Department of Western Australia, 1993; copyright Commonwealth of Australia reproduced by permission)

1. Enjoy a wide variety of nutritious foods.
2. Eat plenty of breads and cereals (preferably wholegrain), vegetables, legumes and fruits.
3. Maintain a diet low in fat and in particular low in saturated fat.
4. Maintain a healthy body weight by balancing physical activity and food intake.
5. If you drink alcohol, limit your intake.
6. Eat only a moderate amount of sugars and foods containing added sugars.
7. Choose low-salt foods and use salt sparingly.
8. Encourage and support breastfeeding.
9. Eat foods containing calcium.
10. Eat foods containing iron.

If you are still unsure as to what these nutritious foods are, here's a simple list to help.

AUSTRALIAN GUIDE TO DAILY FOOD CHOICES
(copyright Commonwealth of Australia reproduced by permission)

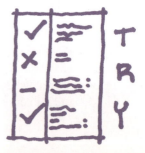

1. 2–3 serves of dairy, yoghurt, milk and cheese
2. 2–3 serves of meat, poultry, fish, dry beans, eggs and nuts (proteins)
3. 2–4 serves of fruit
4. 3–5 serves of vegetables

5. 6–11 serves of bread, cereals, rice and pasta (grains)
6. Eat fats/oils and sweets sparingly

OKINAWAN GUIDELINES (FROM *THE OKINAWA WAY*)
1. Up to 7 servings of meat, poultry and eggs per week
2. 2–4 servings of calcium foods per day
3. 2–4 servings of fruit per day
4. 2–4 servings per day of flavonoid foods, such as soy products, tofu and tempeh
5. 1–3 servings per day of omega-3 foods, such as fish and nuts (walnuts, almonds)
6. Maximum of 3 servings per week of sweets—try to reduce sweet intake and substitute with healthy alternatives, such as fruits with low-fat toppings
7. 1–2 tablespoons per day of vegetable oils and condiments
8. 7–13 servings per day of vegetables, such as broccoli, carrots, peas and so on . . . variety makes our food more interesting
9. 7–13 servings per day of wholegrains, such as rice, noodles and breads

A diet that has lots of vegetables and legumes (especially flavonoids) will help to reduce free-radical damage. Free-radical damage is caused by compounds produced during normal metabolism, as well as by a polluted atmosphere and our busy lifestyles. Research has shown that free radicals can increase our risk of heart disease, cancer, muscular degeneration and dementia. Maintaining a high intake of antioxidants, exercising regularly, and not over-eating may help to reduce the damage caused by free radicals.

Flavonoids

Flavonoids are a type of antioxidant found in a variety of foods, and almost all plant foods, and they are one of the key sources to the longevity of the Okinawa people. Flavonoids can be both a protein and carbohydrate source. Research has shown that the presence of antioxidants in foods can help to reduce the risk of cancer.

Foods high in flavonoids include:

- soy products such as tofu, miso, soybeans and tempeh;
- beans and legumes;
- vegetables such as bok choy, kale, lettuce, onions, celery and carrot tops;
- fruits such as avocados, cherries, cranberries, plums;
- wholegrains such as flaxseed;
- arrowroot, green tea and jasmine tea.

Healthy foods will also help us to maintain strong bones, and even keep our minds sharp by ensuring that clean arteries allow blood circulation to the brain!

A lot of people used to believe that putting on weight as we age is acceptable. We should not gain weight as we age. Gaining weight can increase the risk of all the diseases mentioned above.

If we want to have lean and fit bodies (this means having healthy body fat levels), then we also need to maintain a high level of physical activity.

FLUIDS AND WATER

As mentioned above, water is an essential dietary need. You should aim to consume about 2 litres of fluid a day. You can get fluids from tap water, mineral water, spring water, herbal teas, fruit juices (try to juice them yourself or dilute others) and soups. If that's too hard to work out, then drink enough fluids to ensure your urine is clear in colour and remember to drink even more if you exercise.

ALCOHOL

When you drink alcohol, your liver goes into overdrive. The liver is the emperor of all organs. Its job is to filter and screen any nasty substances coming into the body, and alcohol is just that. Alcohol is a high-energy fuel source, almost as high as fat, but, unlike with fat, the body has no capacity to store alcohol for later use. Therefore the body will burn alcohol first to obtain its energy in preference to all other fuel sources. If the body is using the alcohol as energy, it will store any other sources for future use. That is why people who drink alcohol and eat a lot often gain weight. So you could be packing on the weight just through drinking.

Alcohol is broken down in the body and comes out via the breath, sweat and urine. The liver, however, is responsible for the majority of its processing. In a healthy individual, alcohol is cleared from the bloodstream via the liver at an approximate rate of 5 grams per hour. One standard drink contains approximately 10 grams of alcohol—the equivalent to one middy of beer (285 ml), one 120-ml glass of wine, two middies of light beer, one nip of spirits (30 ml) or 60 ml of port or sherry. So the next time you drink, ask yourself how you are going to burn it off. Do I really need to drink so much or can I sensibly enjoy my drink in moderation?

Studies have shown that the highest level of euphoria a person achieves when drinking alcohol is at the tipsy two- to three-drink stage. At this point, the person is relaxed and they begin to make a couple of mistakes when speaking, such as a stumble or slur here or there. The person is also still aware and they are actually quite amused by their own behaviour. This is the best they are going to get all night. If they continue to drink alcohol, they will find themselves slowly coming down from this peak towards a low level of depression, which can sometimes turn into sadness or aggression. (If the person were to continue to drink indefinitely, their body would eventually lapse into coma.)

If you are aware of this tipsy stage, you can stop drinking for a while and drink some water (alcohol is diuretic, which dehydrates the body) to allow yourself to maintain the euphoric level without putting the body into a downward spiral.

A moderate amount of alcohol, such as two glasses of red wine a night with a couple of alcohol-free days a week, can be good for us. The benefits include decreasing stress and helping to prevent heart disease. A general rule of thumb is one drink a day for women and up to two drinks a day for men is more than enough. Beyond this, the health benefits are outweighed by the adverse effects of alcohol on the body.

TEA AND COFFEE

Tea and coffee (and most chocolates) contain caffeine which stimulates your nervous system, increasing your concentration and focus. However, if you consume too much caffeine, you start to overload your nervous system and consequently find it hard to unwind—you will hold onto your stress more.

A lot of research has been done into the beneficial effects of some Chinese teas—in medicinal terms, they are a source of flavonoids and help to ease digestion and the metabolism of fats. However, all teas, even green teas, still contain caffeine.

As in all dietary needs, moderation is the key to how much caffeine you should have. The best teas in health terms are jasmine, green and oolong. Coffee is okay but limit its intake to one a day, as it does not have as many medicinal values as teas.

TIPS FOR GOOD EATING

Many of us complain that we do not have the time to prepare the exquisite dishes that we like to eat. But you don't have to be a gourmet chef with apprentices on hand to create good food. The most important element is planning. If you spend half an hour thinking about your meals for the week, your life will be filled with a healthy range of foods that will keep you at a peak level, making you feel better, look better and enjoy life more!

Sometimes it is simply good to ask, 'What have I been eating lately? What did I have for breakfast, lunch and dinner?' This can help to encourage you to do something to ensure that you are nourishing and supporting your body with good food by creating opportunities for variety.

Plan three or four major meals in your week, that way you can ensure you write down the ingredients on your shopping list. Allow for leftovers, so that you can have them for lunch the next day or when you can't be bothered cooking. Try to shop monthly for stocks of foods that can be kept for a while, such as dried fruits, pastas, grains and pulses, so you've always got something in the cupboard to use.

Using a journal can help you to look at your current eating habits. Do it for at least one week and make sure you record every meal, every snack, every beer and coffee. Write down how the foods made you feel—you will soon notice that you gravitate towards certain foods in different emotional states. You can then ask yourself if you really needed the food or did it just satisfy a craving. Does satisfying your craving work? Or does it perpetuate the emotions?

You might also want to consider how you eat. The best practices include eating slowly, chewing your food well—working those jaw muscles aids digestion—not skipping meals, and eating smaller, regular meals.

I met an interesting chap who said there was no way that he could possibly alter his lifestyle, especially when it came to business functions that involved alcohol, large meals and smoking. Drinking with clients or friends does not have to be a riotous gorge or a teetotal affair. If we are aware of the food we consume and its effects, we will be in a better position to do something about the way we want to spend our lives and how healthy we want to be.

Ask yourself if you are hungry before you eat. Put down the cutlery every now and then while eating to evaluate how you feel. Take your time, chew your food, be aware, enjoy your meal, don't rush, and try not to do anything else. Unconscious eating can often lead to overeating since you are not paying attention to what you have just consumed and may continue to eat. Taking time to eat and enjoying the sensations and atmosphere of eating can help you to reduce your intake without reducing your enjoyment.

WHAT TO HAVE IN THE KITCHEN

A pantry stocked with good, healthy food means that you won't go looking for fast-food, high-fat alternatives. You will always have something good to eat on hand. Here are some suggestions for your kitchen cupboards (the following list is from *The Okinawa Way*):

OILS
- good quality cold-pressed oils, such as virgin olive oil
- sesame or sunflower oils
- olive oil spray (to reduce the amount of oil you use)

Oils should be kept in dark bottles as they can go rancid when exposed to air and light. You can often use stocks to substitute for oils in your cooking.

FLAVOURS AND SPICES

- vinegars—balsamic, brown rice, white
- rice wine—one good bottle each of red and white
- arrowroot (kuzu)—has medicinal values and acts as a thickener
- turmeric
- curry powder
- basil
- coriander
- rosemary
- bay leaf
- lemons
- oregano
- pepper
- paprika
- sea salt for cooking, not for adding to food at the table
- mustard
- ginger
- chilli
- soy sauce
- vegetable stocks
- sea vegetables—nori, wakame, kombu (dried seaweed)

GRAINS, BEANS, PULSES, NUTS AND SEEDS

- white and brown rice
- barley
- buckwheat
- oats

- breads, preferably made from yeast-free ingredients, such as cornbread, rice cakes, sourdough, essence breads (sprouted breads)
- beans—adzuki, black, chickpeas, lentils, soybean products, broad beans, pinto, kidney
- nuts and seeds—almonds, walnuts, hazelnuts, pumpkin, sesame, sunflower
- wholegrain flour
- soy flour
- wholewheat pasta
- soy nuts (roasted soybeans)
- noodles

TINNED/BOTTLED FOOD
- tomatoes
- vegetables (corn, beetroot, baked beans, artichokes etc.)
- low-fat soups, especially chunky vegetable ones
- fish—tuna, salmon, sardines
- tomato-based pasta sauces (avoid those with preservatives)
- curry pastes (avoid those with preservatives)

FROZEN FOODS
- wholegrain breads
- peas and other vegetables
- low-fat meals

CEREALS
- wholegrain cereals low in fat and sugar

BUY WHEN NEEDED
- tofu/tempeh
- low-fat milk, soy milk or rice milk
- miso (fermented soy bean product), white
- low-fat spreads such as hommus

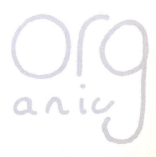

- free-range eggs
- fruit and vegetables in season

Fruit and vegetables in season not only taste better but contain more nutrients. So always try to look for what's in season, not what's been in cold storage. Organic shops usually only stock fruit and vegetables in season, so if in doubt have a look there.

COOKING HINTS

How you prepare and cook your food also impacts on the nutritional value of food. Try the following hints:

MEAT/CHICKEN/FISH
- Trim all visible fat from meat and remove skin from chicken.
- Grill, microwave, barbecue, steam, casserole, stir-fry with stock, or roast the meat on a rack—marinating before cooking can keep the meat tender and moist.
- Avoid frying fish in fat—try wrapping in aluminium foil with a little lemon juice, tomato and herbs or spices and bake in the oven or barbecue. Dip fish in low-fat milk, egg white and breadcrumbs and then bake or dry fry.

OILS/MARGARINES
Use small amounts of any margarine or oil labelled polyunsaturated or mono-unsaturated. Try fat-reduced or 'lite' spreads for sandwiches and toast (not suitable for cooking).

VEGETABLES/SALADS
The bulkier you chop your vegetables, the more your mouth has to work, and the less you will eat. Pre-mixed salad packages can save crucial time for those on the run and are easier to take to work or on your adventures.

- Steam, microwave or boil vegetables in small amounts of water.
- For roast vegetables, steam or microwave first, then brush with a little oil or soy sauce and bake; add seeds and spices for a little flavour.
- When browning, for example onion or stir-frying vegetables, use a little water, stock or unsweetened fruit juice.
- For salad dressings, try lemon juice, low-fat yoghurt, buttermilk, tomato paste, ricotta cheese, mustard, fruit pulp, herbs or vinegar, or use low-calorie commercial salad dressings, such as those with 'no oil'.

Eating out without guilt

When eating out, simply avoid deep-fried foods, creamy and coconut sauces, excessive cheese and battered foods. Lean towards grilled, steamed or barbecued lean meats, vegetables and salads.

Remember

You don't have to have three big meals a day. As long as you maintain your energy levels with healthy snacks through the day, you will be getting all the nutritional requirements you need. Most people tend to have a light breakfast, a light lunch and heavy dinner. I know it can be hard to make time for a good big breakfast, but, if you can start your day with a healthy meal, you are less likely to gorge on sweets around morning-tea time.

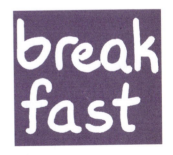

A big meal at dinner is fine if it's early in the evening—the later you eat, the more likely you will go to bed with a full stomach, which often makes it harder to sleep; and you won't be using the energy you have consumed.

FORGOTTEN WHAT TO EAT?

This diagram will get you back on track.

Proteins
- Meat, poultry, fish
- Nuts, eggs
- Legumes, beans and pulses (can eat larger amounts)

Contains: iron, protein, B vitamins (especially B12), zinc, magnesium and omega-3 in fish

Calcium foods
- Low-fat milk products
- Low-fat calcium enriched rice/soy milks
- Low-fat yoghurt and cheeses

Contains: calcium, zinc, proteins, vitamins B12, B2, A and D

Carbohydrates
- Grain products
- Whole grain cereals, pasta, rice, oats
- Noodles, breads (whole grain preferred)

Contains: some calcium, iron, fibre, B vitamins (especially B12)

Fruit, vegetables and legumes
- Dark green leafy vegies
- Orange/yellow vegies
- Beans and pulses
- Lentils, chick peas, soya beans
- Fruits

Contains: vitamins A and C, carotenes, folate, fibre, some carbohydrates

Drink lots of fluids containing water
Small amounts of essential fats from low-fat oils and spreads
Iron sources   Best sources: meats, fish, eggs. Other sources: breads and cereals, beans and pulses, spinach, broccoli, green peas, nuts, seeds and apricots

RECOMMENDED READING

A well-balanced nutritious diet will not only help you look and feel better, but it will also help improve your longevity. In this little book, we have just touched on some of the most accessible ways to improve your health, but, if you are serious about your longevity, I encourage you to read further about the various ways to improve your longevity through nutrition. In particular, have a look at *The Okinawa Way*, to find out more about the healthiest diet in the world.

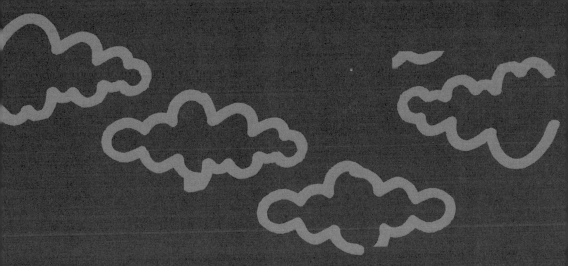

CHAPTER 5

FITNESS FUN

Achieving a healthy level of fitness is not as difficult as you imagine. If we let the body go, life becomes a battle. Simple activities such as walking can become a major feat, mobility is lost, and strength, endurance and spirit sink. An unfit person is likely to gain weight, increase their blood pressure, run the risk of heart disease, and their muscles will start to deteriorate. Other health issues such as high stress levels, diabetes, insomnia, depression, back problems and mental health problems may also develop. Here are some points worth noting:

- Check with your doctor and ensure you get a medical check-up before commencing any of the exercises in this book.
- You don't have to exercise like a gym junkie or marathon runner to become healthy, you just need to be physically active—the more active you are, the fitter and healthier you are.
- You can use your body anywhere and anytime—at work, at home or on the road.
- If you have fun using your body, it's not going to feel like hard work and you will want to do it more and more.
- The more active you become, the fitter and healthier you will become.
- A healthy body increases longevity, and improve quality of life and self-esteem.
- An investment of time need only be as small as two per cent of your day.
- Age is not a limitation!

WITHOUT YOUR BODY YOU CANNOT LIVE

Just as you can't live without the mind, you can't live without your body. And your body affects the way you feel—it can lift or sink your spirit. The body is a jewel in the crown of life, so it should be cherished and worshipped.

Most people think that to be a fit and healthy person you need to train for hours at a gym and take up a running or an outdoor training program. The truth is you don't. A healthy level of fitness can be achieved just by walking and using your body more than you do at the moment—being more active with your body. For most people, the simple step of getting rid of the remote control of the television can help them lose weight.

I teach my clients that many of the activities we consider as recreation are in fact an effective form of exercise. However, I also try not to use the word 'exercise' because it scares so many people away from what is just plain simple activity. If you can look for ways to increase your physical activity during the day, you will help to achieve a shift in your life, immediately. Sounds good doesn't it?

Put simply, the more active you are, the more energy you expend and the more fat you burn. By using your muscles and increasing your heart rate, you also help to lower your resting heart rate and reduce your blood pressure. A healthy person walks about 7000 steps a day, compared with an unhealthy person who may walk only about 2000 steps a day. It's not hard to see how just walking more can help to achieve weight loss and fitness. A lot of people don't realise that using the body can not only be fun, but helps you to live longer, feel and look better. It can also improve your response to stress, your metabolism, sleeping habits, concentration and even your libido!

You don't have to be wafer-thin with a rippling set of abdominals to be healthy, you just need to be active.

People who exercise regularly constitute a very small percentage of our population. One of the reasons for this is that a lot of people don't find physical activity interesting. So, if we can find activities that people like to do and discover which exercises we can incorporate into their lives, we'll be onto a winner.

I call a friend of mine Action Max because he always has some activity on the go, whether he is playing golf, surfing, bushwalking or gold-panning in the bush. Some people would not consider these activities to be exercise, yet, when you break them down, they all are. When Max plays golf, he walks fast between his shots, his heart rate goes up and he gets a cardiovascular work-out. When he's surfing, he is working on his muscular endurance— building muscles in his arms, chest and back. When Max goes hiking, he's working his legs and getting a cardiovascular work-out. When he's squatting down swirling his gold pan, he's building muscle in his legs.

Every one of these activities is physical and they help to keep Max fit and healthy, increasing his chances of living a longer life and being more active throughout it. Best of all, Action Max is having fun!

Obviously, playing darts is not going to get us fit and healthy but walking the dog at a quick pace three times a week for 30 minutes will!

Time

Who's got heaps of spare time? Not many people, yet we don't need to exercise for hours upon hours each day to be healthy and fit. Just three half-hour sessions per week is enough. Work it out—a total of one-and-a-half hours amounts to just about two per cent of your available time. If you are even smarter about how you use your body and what activities you do, you can create effective results without feeling like you have been working at it. The fitter and healthier you get, the more you will have fun and the more you will enjoy yourself.

The key to fitness is to incorporate cardiovascular fitness, muscle strengthening and stretching into your life while having fun and making time for it. When you incorporate these activities into your schedule, you will reduce your risk of heart disease, help achieve fat loss, and maintain your strength to keep yourself mobile and active.

Age is not a limitation

Recent studies have shown that resistance training with weights for nursing home residents aged in their nineties brings results. Even at this age, the participants were able to increase their muscle size and strength. For many, this meant being able to throw away the walking stick because their leg strength had improved so much that they did not need support. It's never too late to start to reclaim your physical strength.

My father is a great example of someone who is fit and healthy but not a sports freak. His exercise regime is a ten-minute series of push-ups, stretches and squats every day. A simple yet effective way of getting the body moving, and keeping strength in the body. His cardiovascular work-out is to walk to work a couple of times a week. On the weekend, he usually goes for a bushwalk.

Pretty simple, nothing overly strenuous, and something that interests him. It's easy to see how keeping physically active keeps him fit and healthy while others his age are overweight and sedentary.

I have trained lots of people who are aged in their sixties, seventies and eighties with positive results. They become stronger, they become fitter, they lose weight if overweight and gain weight if underweight. They look younger and feel better, and most importantly their energy levels increase, their ability to engage in physical activities increases and they reclaim their mobility.

KEY TO FITNESS

I always find that if a fitness program is not simple then I won't be able to remember it. So here goes.

To improve our fitness levels, we need to work on the cardiovascular system. This means increasing the heart rate to a faster beat for a certain amount of time. This will lead to reduced blood pressure, resting heart rate and risk of heart disease. Cardiovascular activities include walking, swimming, running, skiing, bicycle riding, paddling, dancing, skipping, boxing.

To improve our strength, which allows movement of joints in the body, we need to work on the muscular system. The more you allow your muscles to atrophy (reduce in size), the less strength, endurance and, ultimately, mobility you will have. When your mobility is reduced, your freedom begins to fade.

To prevent injuries, release stress and help manage pain, we need to do stretching activities. Stretching makes us more flexible by increasing our range of movements.

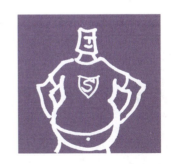

We can't live without air, and the more we use our bodies—walking, running, shovelling or dancing—the more oxygen the body requires to burn fuel to allow us to keep going. This means that when we work the lungs to get more air in and out, the heart pumps more blood around the body.

CARDIOVASCULAR FITNESS

Basically we have three levels of energy that we can work with in cardiovascular fitness:

1. aerobic;
2. lactic acid or anaerobic; and
3. phosphagen or alactic.

A simple way to understand these three energy levels is to look at what type of athlete they serve:

1. aerobic—the distance runner;
2. lactic acid or anaerobic—the 400-metre runner;
3. phosphagen or alactic—the 100-metre sprinter.

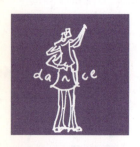

If we look at these distinctly different athletes, we realise that each of them has a specific energy requirement to give them their fuel for their particular event. Yet we all use one fuel—ATP (adenosine triphosphate). ATP provides energy to allow our muscles to slide over each other, allowing movement at a joint. We naturally have about 75 grams of this in the body. But this amount isn't going to last long—we may be able to sprint for about fifteen seconds before we run out of this fuel. We have enough ATP to help us in an emergency situation but when it's all gone, we have to recombine it to allow us to keep going.

In order to replenish our stores of ATP, we need to use one of the three energy levels.

AEROBIC
The most effective energy level for weight/fat loss is aerobic. This is also what the endurance (distance) athlete uses—whether they are doing a triathlon, or a half-hour walk at a brisk pace.

With aerobic activity, oxygen is distributed throughout the body via the blood. In its presence, carbohydrates are burnt to provide energy, which replenishes our stores of ATP for us to use over and over.

Training with this system helps to develop your slow twitch muscle fibres (see 'Muscle work-out' below for an explanation of slow twitch and fast twitch muscle fibres), target fat loss, increase your cardiac output (blood pumped through the body), reduce your blood pressure and lower your resting heart beat. These athletes are generally lean with a very defined muscle structure. To achieve the best results with the aerobic energy system, you need to train (run, swim, walk, cycle) at a certain intensity.

Level of intensity relates to your heart rate (HR). To work out the intensity of an activity, you need to gauge what percentage of your maximum heart rate (MHR), your heart is beating at during the activity. This can be as simple as asking yourself, 'How much effort does this feel like—very light, light, somewhat hard, hard, very hard, or extremely hard?' If you describe your intensity as somewhere between light to somewhat hard, then you are exercising at an HR of between 60 and 75 per cent of your MHR. If the intensity is very light, the activity is not, aerobically, very effective. If you are working hard to extremely hard, you have shifted into the lactic acid or anaerobic energy level.

LACTIC ACID OR ANAEROBIC

Exercising at an HR of between 75 and 85 per cent of your MHR means that you are working at a lactic acid or anaerobic energy level. If you work-out for longer than 60 seconds at this intensity, you will experience a build-up of lactic acid in your body and you are going to fatigue. At this intensity, you are using up ATP faster than it can be replenished by aerobic activity. The only option your body has is to break down glycogen/glucose to provide the energy to recombine ATP. The problem with this system is the by-product of lactic acid—its levels get too high and our muscles fatigue.

This energy system is what 400-metre runners use. It targets cardiac output, fast and slow twitch muscle fibres and blood pressure.

Phosphagen (creatine phosphate) or alactic

When exercising at an HR of between 85 and 95 per cent of your MHR, you use the phosphagen or alactic energy system. You only have about ten to fifteen seconds available at this intensity.

This energy system is fuelled by phosphagen (creatine phosphate), which is stored in small amounts within each cell. The phosphate molecule is broken down to provide energy to recombine the ATP. When the stores of phosphagen are exhausted, the next energy system kicks in—the slower lactic acid energy system. The 100-metre sprinter uses this energy, which targets the fast twitch muscle fibres, cardiac output and blood perfusion.

You are unique both in body and mind. Your body has its own proportion of fast and slow twitch muscle fibres. When most of us start training, we have the urge to run at full pace and collapse. But, if you know which energy system you want to target, you can just stick to the intensity level for that energy system.

Sprinters have a higher proportion of fast twitch muscle fibres, which means their muscles contract quickly. A higher percentage of fast twitch fibres is found in sports with quick or strong movements. Endurance athletes, on the other hand, have a higher proportion of slow twitch muscle fibres. Some of us have a more balanced proportion. This can help to explain why we find some types of training more fun than others.

If, for example, you have a higher proportion of fast twitch fibres, you may find you prefer to do sprints rather than a long slow jog. Or perhaps you like to lift heavy weights. When we practise training at the different energy levels, we soon find out which activities we prefer and to which our body is more suited.

The hardest thing you will find when training is to start at the intensity you are at. A classic example which I see on the streets is the middle-aged bloke going for a run. He hopes to lose his beer gut through some exercise and decides to go for the most intense physical activity we can put the body through—running.

After donning the footy guernsey and old trainers, he starts to sprint down the street—he will have just gone straight into the phosphagen energy system. Within fifteen seconds, he will be fatiguing, then slowing down and starting to use the lactic energy system. After 60 seconds, he will feel he can't run a step more at that pace without collapsing. His body fatigues and he feels all the effects that an Olympic athlete feels after their 400-metre run. He starts to walk and feels dejected, unfit, sick, and will have only made it halfway around the block. After a couple of minutes, he may try again, but, once again, at an intensity much harder than required for his target (fat loss). After making it around the block, he goes home vowing to never exercise again. Who could blame him with the fatigue he would be feeling?

I believe that much of the population just wants to target fat loss, to look and feel good about themselves, and increase their longevity. The best way to achieve this is to use the FITT principle:

Frequency: 3–5 times per week
Intensity: light to somewhat hard
Type: an activity that moves the large muscle groups of the body i.e. not thumb wrestling!
Time: 20–40 minutes.

Frequency
Intensity
Time
Type

Remember, you can choose any fun activity that comes to mind as long as it uses the large muscle groups. So, if you head out at night and dance for half an hour, you have just fulfilled one of the three sessions per week you need for cardiovascular fitness.

Sometimes, 30 minutes may be just too much to find. In these situations, three ten-minute sessions will help to achieve the same result. This could be a brisk walk to the train station in the morning, a ten-minute walk at lunch time to the city park during a work day, followed in the evening by a brisk ten-minute walk with the dog.

For some, a weekly golf game can provide one session, but just make sure you drink a mineral water and not a beer after the game. Perhaps you can walk to a work meeting, or to the post office and local shop? Obviously, if you do the same thing all the time, you might get bored! If you can cross-train and change the pace, then you will enjoy the benefits of all energy levels while having a lot more fun!

One way you can do this is to exercise within your aerobic energy zone (light to somewhat hard intensity), mixed with five minutes of lactic acid energy (maximum 60 seconds at hard to very hard), adding a topping of two minutes of the phosphagen energy system (maximum ten seconds at very hard to extremely hard). You can combine this any way you like. If it's fat loss you're after, always include 30 minutes of the aerobic energy system.

MUSCLE WORK-OUT

Everyone has muscles, not just body builders. Just by reading this book you are using muscles in your eyes, forearms, hands and neck. If we stop and think about which muscles we use in our daily activities, we can see what we need to focus on to keep our bodies working well. For example, if you sit at a desk when working, your abdominal muscles could waste away and you are much more likely to get back pain, so you need to work on your abdominals in other activities.

If the number of muscles you use is very limited, then your muscles will slowly reduce in size, causing reduced mobility.

We have a combination of both slow twitch and fast twitch muscle fibres in our bodies. Those with a higher proportion of slow twitch muscle fibres are suited to endurance events, and those with fast twitch are more suited to sprinting events.

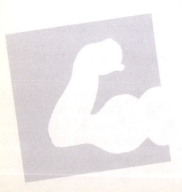

When we are young, we have more fast twitch muscle fibres. As we age, we come to recognise which type we have more of by what we are capable of doing. So there is a reason why you may perform well over short distances but fall way behind in longer distances.

The 'large muscle groups', as referred to in the FITT principle, include the back, legs and chest muscles. The other main muscles in the body are the shoulders, abdominals and arms. The bigger the muscle, the more oxygen you need for the aerobic energy system to operate, which means you require more fuels in the form of carbohydrates, proteins or fats.

Weight training

We don't have to lift weights in order to achieve the muscular strength that we need to remain healthy and mobile, but we do need to do weight-bearing excercises. Of course, if you can lift weights and can tailor a program to achieve what you want, that's great, but most of us will do just as well if we perform the right amounts of weight-bearing exercises.

Ask yourself: What do I want to achieve? Is it fat loss, bigger muscles or stronger muscles? If you want fat loss but don't want to get any bigger, muscular endurance will give you lean and toned muscles. Muscular hypertrophy will give you the biggest muscles possible, and muscular strength gives you the strongest but not the biggest muscles. The actual weight you lift depends on which result you want.

Repetition maximum (RM) is the maximum weight you could lift only once. For example, if I tried to lift 100 kilograms and I couldn't do it, then my RM would be lower than that, so I would try a lighter weight to see if I could lift it. It isn't necessary to lift every weight trying to find your RM. It can be estimated with a little bit of practice, starting with a light weight.

Always seek professional advice when weight training and never try to lift heavy weights without the right supervision. It's imperative that you learn how to lift weights safely before proceeding on your own.

A very common question about weight training is spot reduction. For example, 'If I do heaps of sit-ups, can I get rid of my gut and get a "six-pack"?'

Unfortunately, the answer here is no. If we look at a professional tennis player's arms, we can see why. They use one arm all the time, the other one doesn't do much at all. The muscle size on the playing arm is huge compared to the other arm, but, when we measure the fat content of each arm, they are exactly the same. So, even if we work out on a particular point in the body, we may be able to develop the muscle but we will not necessarily target the fat.

Fat is stored in different areas of the body. Women store fat around the buttocks and thighs, while men tend to store it around the stomach. If you want to target fat loss, you need to look at a general aerobic work-out or overall weight training program to achieve results. Doing an abdominal work-out in conjunction with a weight training program or aerobic work-out, will help because you will be burning fuel and energy, and you will have less fat to store on the body.

STRETCHING MOVEMENTS

Stretching makes us stronger by increasing our range of movement. Stretching is natural, it's just that most of us have lost this connection with our bodies. We may do it now and then, such as a neck stretch after straining on the computer or reading a book, or a back stretch after leaning over all day. But the importance of stretching is always underestimated. Stretching relaxes the mind, prevents injury, improves circulation, increases range of movement through joints, releases stress and helps to manage pain.

When we stretch, we develop awareness of what keeps the body together; we also find out what we have been ignoring, and where the body shows tension, stress or pain. After we stretch we feel invigorated, peaceful and, most importantly, our muscles and joints are ready to keep working with greater range and less risk of injury.

Below we have listed some key stretches to help you stay out of trouble. Before you begin any stretching, it is important that you make sure you warm up sufficiently to minimise any possible muscle strain or injury. Check with your doctor if you are worried about any particular condition before commencing any of the stretching exercises. To warm up, you can begin by walking on the spot and moving your arms for a few of minutes.

We will look at each of these in more detail later on in this chapter. See the 'Stretch class' on page 84.

Chest	Back and triceps	Legs—Hamstrings
Wrists	Legs—Quadriceps	Lower back
Shoulders	Legs—Calves	Back—Cat stretch

Make it a part of your life

We live in the technological age where everything is designed to make things easier for us physically. If we can put our bodies back into the equation, we can start expending more energy, burning more fuel and fat, and help to maintain muscles.

There is a huge list of activities you can choose from to develop fitness in the workplace and in everyday life. The more opportunities you take to use your body, the more you can burn energy.

Everyday life

Just look around! Everywhere you go there is a smorgasbord of activities waiting to help you to be more active and become fitter. Consider the following simple steps towards a healthier lifestyle:

- walk, cycle or roller blade to work;
- get rid of the television remote control;
- run for the bus;
- take the stairs instead of the elevator;
- do some gardening;
- walk/run the dog;
- go for a scenic sightseeing walk;
- walk home from the restaurant;
- carry the shopping bags to the car instead of using a trolley;
- use a child backpack rather than a stroller;

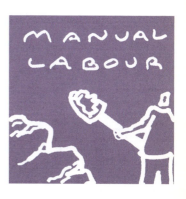

- ride a pushbike;
- hang on to some branches then swing upside down;
- go to the playground and swing on the monkey bars, climb the ladders or use the swings;
- play games with the kids and see how quickly you tire—a real work-out!;
- train with a sports team;
- help coach the kids' sports team;
- walk and do some lunges every now and then;
- run down the street at full pace, just to see what it feels like (avoid running into people by ducking and weaving—an added bonus);
- walk/run backwards and sideways (use a smooth surface so you don't trip over);
- walk on all fours (hands and feet);
- bound like a rabbit or jump like a frog.

If you're doing something fun and you love it, it's not going to feel like work at all. If you like tennis, then play it. If you're into golf, then have a game (just make sure you put in a brisk walk and avoid drinks at the clubhouse). If you like hiking, walk briskly so you get a better result. All you have to do to increase physical activity is to think about how you can increase the toll that you put on your body. For example, 'If I walk faster, the body will work harder.'

Sometimes it's good to work on things that are different to your nature. If you're passive, it's good to do an active sport; if you are very active, do a pacifying activity such as Tai Chi or yoga.

Dancing is a fun way to get fit and meet new people or involve a partner. Just try to avoid alcohol if you are out on the town. Consider linedancing, salsa or ballroom dancing.

Team sports can be a great way to get fit. There are heaps to choose from, such as touch football, volleyball, soccer—any team activity that involves aerobic conditioning.

If you want to get fit and in touch with the environment, try hiking/bushwalking, orienteering, canoeing, kayaking, cross-country skiing, golf or wind surfing.

Fitness activities for the more adventurous include rock climbing, surfing, mountain biking, whitewater kayaking, rafting, kite surfing, snowboarding and skiing. Water activities, such as aquarobics, swimming and diving, are also good fun.

If you are recovering from injuries, there are therapeutic activities such as hydrotherapy, yoga and pilates.

'Domestic chores', such as gardening, labouring, shovelling, lifting with bent knees and handwashing the car, all help towards your goals.

Yoga and martial arts, such as kung fu, karate or tae kwon do, are active forms that require discipline and focus, which is great for mind and body. More defensive forms include judo, jujitsu and capoeira.

Acrobatics and gymnastics are other fun ways to get fit and have a good time while doing it.

THE OFFICE GYMNASIUM

Even if you work in an office, you can increase your energy expenditure (activity) by squeezing in some traditional exercises to help build and maintain muscle mass. See if you can walk around the office more by moving the printer away from the computer so you have to walk to it. Also, when your energy feels low, take a walk to get some blood moving through your body.

When you are on the telephone take the call on your feet. Simply standing will expend more energy than sitting down.

While getting out of a chair put your hands on the armrests and push down through your arms, trying to take all of your weight in your arms. Once you are up, slowly lower yourself down. Repeat this a few times then get up and go. You have just exercised your tricep and shoulder muscles.

Walk down the corridor doing some lunges. You might get some weird looks from your colleagues, but you'll be getting a good work-out! To lunge, take a long step forward with one leg, bending your knee towards the floor. Keep your other leg firmly in place, straight, with your heel pressed into the ground. Make sure you don't bend the front knee more than an angle of 90 degrees. Repeat on the other side. You have just worked your glutes, quadriceps, hamstrings and calves.

Other exercises could include push-ups using the desk to lean on. You can even work out without getting out of the chair—lift your knees to your chest while sitting to work your abdominal muscles.

Just look around and think about all the items you can use—chairs, desks, stairs, door arches—to work the body and expend some energy.

Find some floor space either in the print room or under the desk. You may get a few weird looks but people will often start to try it out themselves and then

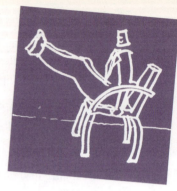

join in. Some of the best exercises we can do in this environment are push-ups, sit-ups, lunges, side leans and chin-ups—if you have strong fingers and a very sturdy door frame (great for rock climbers).

Climb the stairs quickly, one at a time, two at a time, three, or even four if you can. To exercise your calf muscles, stand on the edge of a step with both toes pointing in towards the step but with your heel and middle of your foot hanging over the edge of the step. Inhale as you lower your heel down below the top of the step, and exhale as you push through your toes and take your heels higher than the step. Feel it do its work.

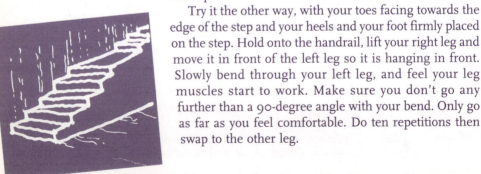

Try it the other way, with your toes facing towards the edge of the step and your heels and your foot firmly placed on the step. Hold onto the handrail, lift your right leg and move it in front of the left leg so it is hanging in front. Slowly bend through your left leg, and feel your leg muscles start to work. Make sure you don't go any further than a 90-degree angle with your bend. Only go as far as you feel comfortable. Do ten repetitions then swap to the other leg.

Investment

You can look at your body as an investment—if I am going to be putting money, effort and time into it, what kind of return am I going to get? If you commit just 30 minutes three times a week, you can lower blood pressure, reduce the risk of heart disease, lower your resting heart rate, reduce your fat levels, and build and maintain your muscle mass. This adds up to only about two per cent of your time.

Your second investment entails using your will and motivation—you really need to make a choice to be healthy. If you are having difficulties, try the 'winter yoga' in Chapter 6 to fire up your motivation. Then follow this with the 'Make a choice in your life to be healthy' and the 'intuition exercise' in Chapter 9.

A healthy body will help you to achieve longevity, and improve your quality of life and self-esteem. If you make no effort, you are likely to gain weight, increase the likehood of diseases and your muscles will start to deteriorate.

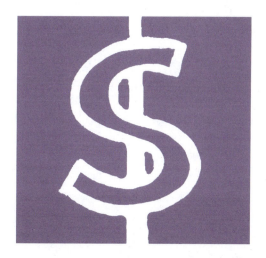

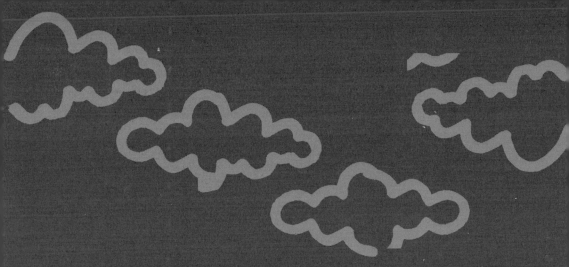

CHAPTER 6

YOGA

- Do you want to look and feel younger?
- Do you want to release pain and tension from your body?
- Do you want to feel energised?
- Do you want to feel emotionally prepared for life?
- Do you want to adapt to changes of the seasons?

The origins of yoga date as far back as three thousand years. Even that long ago, people were looking for ways to help themselves, physically, mentally and spiritually. Yoga to me provides all of these things and more.

I see the body as a machine. It is amazingly crafted, designed and constructed, and the way it works still has us baffled. Yet we abuse it, neglect it and fail to service this vital piece of machinery. If it is not functioning properly, our quality of life declines and our ability to do what we want is affected. Our mobility, drive and motivation deteriorate and we begin the downhill run into the final cycle of our body's existence.

Sounds a bit deep—yet it rings true doesn't it?

As I write the words to this chapter, I am experiencing a downward spiral. Thanks to a mistake I made while hang-gliding I am sporting the injury of a sore and swollen leg with 30 stitches to boot. In a weird way, I appreciate getting injured because I now realise how lucky I am to have my health, fitness and vitality. In the few days since I injured myself, I have discovered all the aches and pains of a body that has not been used. 'Use it or lose it' is a very true statement.

Because I've not been able to use my body, I now have a sore back—and I didn't hurt it flying! I also feel lethargic instead of invigorated, energised and motivated! But I know how to fix the problem and I've learnt my lesson. I will do a yoga session, which will release my back pain and lift my emotions.

Rather than spend pages explaining to you how yoga works, I will give you a simple explanation of how I relate to it. I am sure you have watched little children playing, tumbling, turning, twisting, jumping, rolling, hanging upside down, pushing, pulling, stretching, moving, holding, laying still. Children are a great inspiration and example of what we are trying to achieve when doing yoga and some of the effects of the postures.

Every time a child rolls around in a tumble, they are moving blood around their body and altering the effects of gravity, altering the way blood runs to their heads, and to their other extremities, such as their fingers and toes. They also keep their joints and muscles active, flexible and strong yet not rigid. They thrive on activity and their skin has a vital glow. They do not have problems with digestion. They do not hold tension, and they express themselves with their bodies. Their eyes are bright, clear and healthy. Their spines are supple and flexible, their postures upright and erect. They are healthy, happy and alive.

This is what yoga can do for you. Every time you do an inverted position (one with your legs in the air), you are reversing the effects of gravity. When you move through a posture, you release tension and help the body to release toxins. At the same time, you increase your flexibility and strength, which keeps you strong, moving and coordinated.

Yoga literally means 'union'. It helps you to connect your mind, body and spirit. Yoga involves using lots of tools—asanas (postures), meditation, breathing (pranayama) and more—to achieve this union. I am focusing on the asana (postures) in this chapter. (You will find more on meditation and breathing in other chapters.) Why not try some of the asanas and see how you feel physically, emotionally and spiritually afterwards?

There are no limitations to who can do yoga—if you can breathe, you can do yoga. The benefits are numerous. It can help you to look and feel younger, improve your muscular strength, and release pain and tension from the body. Yoga can also help to improve your sleep, digestion and your sense of purpose in life. The list goes on. In this chapter, we use yoga to address common problems to help maintain your general health.

This series of classes includes asanas for the different meridians (energy channels) which run through the body affecting you both physically and emotionally. There's also a general class of meridians for each season. By considering the meridians, you can choose a class that may relate to a particular emotional or physical problem which you may have. The following pages list each class offered and the corresponding meridians, body parts and emotions that are affected.

Tips

- Exhale through the mouth for dynamic asanas to blow out resistance from the body and mind.
- Only stretch to as far as you feel comfortable.
- If you are pregnant, please find a specialist antenatal yoga class.
- If you have any injuries, check with your doctor or health practitioner to ensure that yoga will not aggravate your injury.
- Always do a back warm-up exercise before commencing any corrective posture exercises.

Summer

Meridians affected—heart, triple heater, heart constrictor, small intestine.

Body parts affected—small intestine, heart, blood pressure and circulation, strength, power.

Emotions affected—power, creativity, joy and inspiration, happiness and sadness.

Late summer and between the seasons

Meridians affected—stomach, spleen.

Body parts affected—stomach, front of the body, thighs, breasts, energy levels.

Emotions affected—awareness, sense of nourishment, desire.

Autumn

Meridians affected—lungs and large intestine.

Body parts affected—colon, lungs, chest, upper back, back of thighs, buttocks.

Emotions affected—vitality, letting go of old emotions, relationships, events, hope, decision making.

WINTER

Meridians affected—kidneys and urinary/bladder.
Body parts affected—bladder, hearing, sense of balance, neck, nervous system.
Emotions affected—motivation, will, drive, confidence, nervousness, ability to deal with stress.

SPRING

Meridians affected—liver, gall bladder.
Body parts affected—gall bladder, liver, joints, ligaments, flexibility, sight, hips, knees, shoulders.
Emotions affected—vision, organisation, responsibility, discipline, flexibility, patience.

PROBLEMS WITH EMOTIONS

Motivation, will, drive, confidence—do a winter (kidneys bladder energy) class
Nervousness, tension—do a winter (bladder energy) class
Swinging emotions (between happiness and sadness for example), sense of joy—do a summer (heart energy) class
Over-organised, disorganised, over- or undisciplined—do a spring (gall bladder energy) class
Holding onto past emotions or events—do an autumn (large intestine energy) class
No sense of what to do in the future, where you are going—do a summer (liver energy) class
Feeling powerless—do a spring (small intestine energy) class
Feeling unsupported and alone—do a late summer (spleen energy) class
Feeling like you have lost your sense of awareness of things around you—do a late summer (stomach energy) class
Not feeling like doing anything, lost your sense of vitality and lightness—do an autumn (lung) class

Not in touch with your environment or the people around you—do a summer (triple heater) class

Feeling disconnected from your body, or as if you are stuck in your head—do a summer (heart constrictor) class

PROBLEMS WITH THE BODY

Sore lower back—do a back and winter (kidneys and bladder) class
Bad hips—do a winter and spring (kidneys and liver energy) class
Sore middle back—do a late summer (spleen) class
Sore upper back (between shoulder blades)—do a spring (gall bladder) class
Sore neck—do a winter and autumn (bladder and lung) class
Headache—do a winter (bladder energy) class
Sciatica—do a winter (bladder) class
Eyesight—do a spring (liver energy) class
Digestion—do a late summer, autumn and summer (stomach, large intestine and small intestine energy) class
Diarrhoea—do an autumn (large intestine) class
Constipation—do an autumn (large intestine) class
Asthma—do an autumn, late summer and winter (lung and large intestine, spleen and kidneys) class
Sore joints, arthritis—do a spring (liver energy) class
Blood pressure—do a summer (heart constrictor energy) class
Cold fingers and toes—do a summer (heart constrictor) class
Tightness in back of legs—do a winter (bladder) class
Stammering—do a summer (heart) class
Colds and flus—do a winter (large intestine) class

If you discover you like yoga, try to find a yoga class nearby—you'll find out what group energy is all about. You will also be able to receive individual attention for any specific problems you have.

STRETCH CLASS

⇨ Stand or kneel, interlock your fingers behind your back with palms facing towards your body and hands resting near your buttocks. Inhale, then exhale as you take your arms away from your buttocks up towards the middle of your back. Push your chest forward to feel the stretch. Hold the stretch for a count of 10, breathing normally.

⇨ Stand with the side of your body parallel to a wall or post, palm resting on the edge of the wall or post. Inhale, then exhale as you push your palm onto the surface. Feel the stretch down through the arm, holding for a count of 10, breathing normally. Repeat on the other side to stretch both arms.

⇨ Stand or kneel, hold your right hand in front of your body, with fingers pointing up, your shoulders relaxed. Inhale, then exhale as you push the heel of your right palm forwards and pull back on the fingertips with your left hand. Hold for a count of 10, breathing normally. Repeat with the left arm.

⇨ Stand or kneel, hold your right hand in front of your body with your fingers pointing down and your palms towards your body. Inhale, then exhale as you push your fingers towards your body, with your left hand. Hold for a count of 10, breathing normally. Repeat with the left arm.

⇨ Take your right arm across your body, inhale, placing your left arm underneath your right elbow. Exhale as you bend your left arm and pull your right arm towards your left shoulder. Hold for a count of 10, breathing normally. Repeat with your left arm.

⇨ Take your right arm behind your head, inhale, placing your left hand on top of your right elbow. Exhale as you take your right elbow across, push down and hold with your left hand. Hold for a count of 10, breathing normally. Repeat with your left arm.

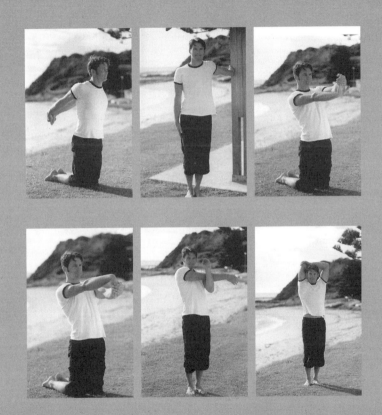

⇨ Stand an arm's length away from a wall or post, rest your left hand on the wall, inhale, then exhale as you hold your right foot with your right hand and lift it up towards your buttocks. Inhale, then as you exhale, squeeze your knees together and pull the back of your foot towards your buttocks. Hold for a count of 10, breathing normally. Repeat with your left leg.

⇨ Stand an arm's length away from a wall, press both hands on the wall, inhale, then exhale, stepping back with your right foot until only your toes and ball of your foot are touching the ground. Inhale, then exhale as you push your heel towards the ground and bend your left knee forward. Feel the stretch in the back of your right calf muscle. Hold for a count of 10, breathing normally. Repeat with your left leg.

⇨ Lay on the ground, your left leg straight on the ground, bend your right knee to your chest to prepare. Hold your leg with both hands from the calves or thighs, not behind the knee, breathe in, then as you exhale, straighten the leg as much as possible. If this is too hard, hold closer to the thighs, if it's too easy, slide your hands towards your foot. Keep your toes pulled back and hold for a count of 10, breathing normally. Repeat with your left leg.

⇨ Interlock your fingers behind your head, elbows wide, your legs bent, feet close to your buttocks, and knees close together. Inhale to prepare. Slowly take your knees to the right, keeping your knees together and exhale as you look towards your left elbow. Don't collapse, hold for a count of 10, breathing normally. Then inhale and move your legs back to centre. Repeat on the other side.

⇨ Rest on all fours with your hands beneath your shoulders, your knees beneath your hips. Inhale to prepare. Exhale as you arch like a cat, dropping your head to look towards your navel, and hold for a count of 10, breathing normally. Inhale and return back to centre. Then exhale as you lower your belly to the ground, looking upwards. Hold for a count of 10, breathing normally. Inhale and return to centre.

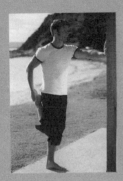
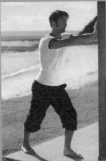
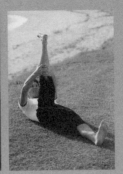

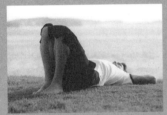
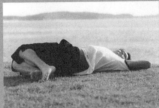
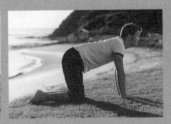

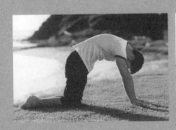
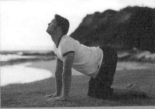

BACK WARM-UP CLASS

⇨ Rest on all fours with your hands beneath your shoulders and your fingers pointing forwards. Inhale to prepare.

⇨ Exhale as you lean forward, taking your weight over your wrists and keeping your arms straight. Inhale to return back to centre. Repeat 5–10 times.

⇨ Turn your fingers back towards your knees, if too difficult turn your fingers out to the sides. Inhale to prepare, then exhale as you take your weight over your wrists, and your buttocks towards your heels. Inhale to return to centre. Repeat 5–10 times.

⇨ Turn your fingers forwards once more. Inhale to bend your knee towards your forehead, arching your back upwards.

⇨ Exhale as you extend your leg behind and upwards, looking upwards with your head. Inhale to bend your knee to your forehead once more. Repeat 10 times.

⇨ Inhale to extend your leg in line with your hips, then exhale as you move your leg across to one side and look over your shoulder at it. Inhale to return to centre and exhale as you move your leg to the other side and look over your shoulder. Inhale to return to centre. Repeat 10 times, then repeat the whole sequence with your other leg.

⇨ Sit with your legs extended in front and your toes pulled back. Inhale and lift out of your chest.

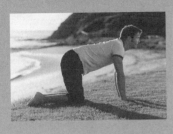
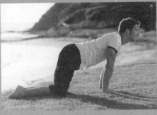
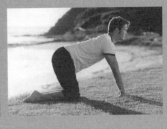

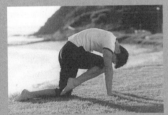
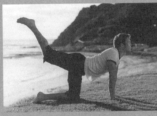
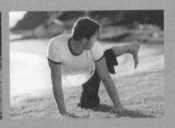

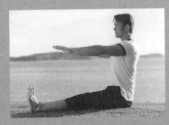
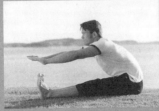
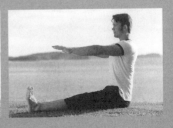

⇨ Exhale as you push forwards from your hips, keeping your toes pulled back.

⇨ Inhale to return to centre. Exhale as you lean halfway back. Repeat the whole sequence 10 times.

⇨ Sit with your buttocks on your heels, your arms stretched forward fingers on the ground. Inhale to prepare.

⇨ As you exhale, move your chest forward, preparing to drape your hips. Inhale as you straighten your arms, lifting your chest away from the floor, and look up, drawing your shoulders away from your ears.

⇨ Exhale as you arch like a cat, head bent, looking at your navel.

⇨ Inhale as you take your buttocks back to your heels and look forward. Repeat the sequence twice.

⇨ Interlock your fingers behind, elbows wide, your legs bent, feet close to your buttocks, and knees close together. Inhale to prepare. Slowly take your knees to the right, keeping your knees together and exhale as you look towards your left elbow. Don't collapse, hold for a count of 10, breathing normally. Then inhale and move your legs back to centre. Repeat on the other side.

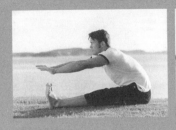 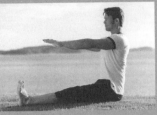 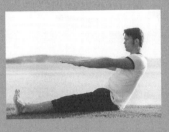

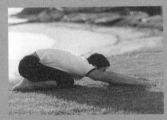 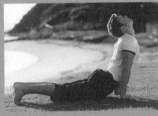 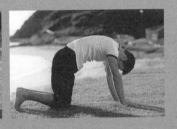

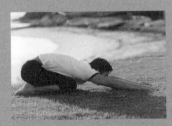 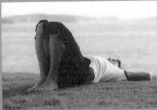 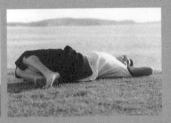

SPRING CLASS (LIVER AND GALL BLADDER ENERGY MERIDIANS)

⇨ Sit in a kneeling position, interlock your fingers above your head with palms facing upwards and inhale.

⇨ Exhale as you move your hips to one side, while pushing your palms up and outwards. Inhale to return to centre and repeat to the other side.

⇨ Kneel on all fours and inhale to prepare. Exhale as you swing your foot from centre to side, looking over your shoulder to your toes. Inhale to return to centre. Repeat on the other side, then repeat 10 times.

⇨ Kneel on all fours and inhale to prepare. Exhale as you move your hips down towards the ground without collapsing. Inhale to return to centre. Repeat on the other side.

⇨ Lie on your left side, legs extended, arms along your sides. Inhale to lift both legs and curl up the side of your torso at the same time. Exhale as you slowly come down, keeping the tension on your side and belly, inhale, and repeat 10 times, then repeat on the other side.

⇨ Lie on your left side, prop up your torso with your forearm, inhale to take your right leg over in front of your left leg, then exhale to lift your left leg. Inhale to take your leg down and repeat 10 times, then repeat on the other side.

⇨ Lie on the ground, legs extended, with your feet together, toes pulled back, arms out at 90 degrees and palms facing the ground. Inhale to prepare. Exhale as you lift your right leg up vertically, keeping your toes pulled back and your tail bone anchored to the ground.

⇨ Inhale, then exhale as you move your right leg over to the left side and look towards your right hand.

⇨ Inhale as you move your leg back to vertical, then exhale as you move your leg to the right side, looking towards your left hand. Repeat on the other leg.

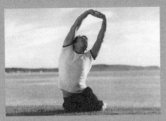 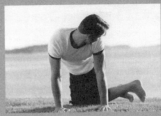 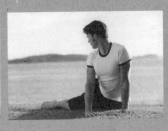

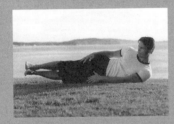 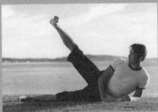 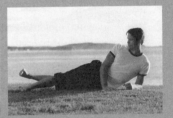

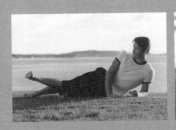 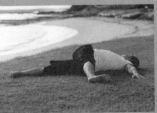 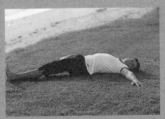

⇨ Sit with your legs long and wide, your toes pulled back, your hands behind your head, and inhale.

    Move your chest forward as you exhale, keeping your toes pulled back. Inhale to return to centre.

⇨ Remaining in the above position, your hands behind your head, inhale to bring your left elbow in front of your left knee, stretching long on your other side. Exhale and look up at your right elbow. Inhale to return to centre. Repeat on the other side; repeat 10 times.

⇨ Sit with your legs wide, inhale to take your left elbow in front of your left knee and hold onto your big toe with your left hand if possible. Exhale as you extend your right arm over, taking your right hand close to your left foot, hold for 3 breaths, inhale to return to centre. Repeat on the other side.

⇨ Sit with your legs wide and your toes pulled back. Inhale to prepare.

    Exhale as you twist to one side, and place both arms behind you. Inhale to return to centre, then exhale to twist to the other side.

⇨ Lie on your back with your right arm at a right angle to your torso, your palm facing downwards. Inhale to lift your right foot near your left knee. Exhale as you move your right knee down to your left side, and look towards your right hand. Hold this pose for 5–10 breaths. Inhale to return to centre and repeat on the other side.

⇨ Rest pose: Lie on your back, legs and arms extended, palms facing up, feet flopped out to the sides.

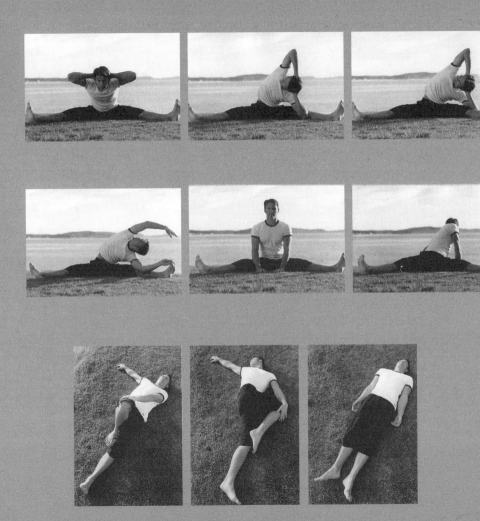

SUMMER CLASS (HEART AND HEART CONSTRICTOR ENERGY, SMALL INTESTINE AND TRIPLE HEATER MERIDIANS)

⇨ Sit with your buttocks resting on your heels. Rub vigorously up and down the side of your arm, the back of your triceps, then down your forearm until you feel warm. Then squeeze down the side of your hand. Repeat on the other side.

⇨ Take your right arm behind your head, inhale to place your left hand on top of your elbow. Exhale as you take your right elbow across, and hold for 5–10 breaths. Inhale to relax to centre and repeat on the other side.

⇨ Tuck your thumbs into fists and inhale to bring your elbows together. Exhale as you thrust your hips forward, lifting away from your heels, and take your arms out to the side. Inhale and sit back down. Repeat 5–10 times.

⇨ Take your right arm behind your head and try to join your hands behind your back, or grab your shirt. Inhale to pull back your right elbow. Exhale as you thrust your hips forward, lifting away from your heels, pulling back on your right elbow. Inhale and slowly sit down. Repeat 5–10 times, then repeat with your left arm.

⇨ Lie on your back, interlock fingers behind your head. Bring knees up with feet close to buttocks, keeping knees together. Inhale to prepare. Exhale as you slowly take your knees to the right side, looking towards your left elbow, making sure not to collapse. Inhale to return to centre and repeat on the other side. Repeat 5–10 times.

⇨ Lie on your back, lifting your legs to right angles, so that your calves are parallel to the ground. Inhale and squeeze your knees together. Exhale as you slowly move your knees to the right side, looking towards your left elbow, making sure not to collapse. Inhale to return to centre and repeat on the other side. Repeat 5–10 times.

⇨ Lie on your back, bringing your knees as close to your chest as possible. Inhale and squeeze your knees together. Exhale as you slowly move your knees to the right side, looking towards your left elbow, making sure not to collapse. Inhale to return to centre and repeat on the other side. Repeat 5–10 times.

⇨ Sit with legs as wide as possible, tuck thumbs into fists and place them under armpits. Inhale to lift out of your chest. Exhale as you lean forward, keeping chin tucked in, and your toes pulled back. Inhale to return to centre and repeat 5–10 times.

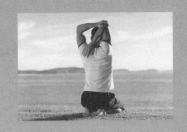
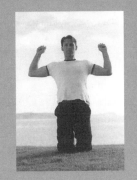
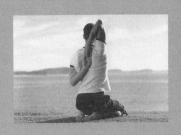

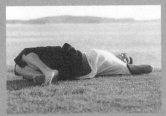
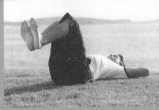
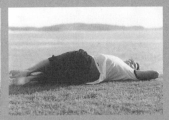

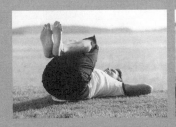
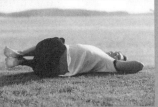
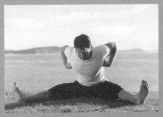

⇨ Lie on your belly, your hands close to your chest, with your fingers pointing forwards. Inhale to prepare. Squeeze your elbows together as you exhale and try to come up halfway into a push-up. Inhale to return to the ground. (This is a difficult movement, but if you can take it further, try it with straight legs.) Repeat 5 times.

⇨ Remaining on your belly, inhale and squeeze your elbows together, exhale as you push up. Hold the position as you inhale and rock forwards, then exhale to rock backwards, until you are out of breath. Try to rock a few more times, remembering to breathe, then rest.

⇨ Lie on your belly with your legs just wider than hip width, toes dug into the ground. Your right arm is out to the side, and your left hand is above your head. Inhale to prepare. Exhale as you take your right arm into a vertical position, keeping your knees on the ground. Flex your hand and stretch through your middle finger. Inhale to bring your arm down. Repeat 5 times.

⇨ Remaining in the above position, inhale to prepare, then exhale as you take your right arm as far over as possible, keeping your knees on the ground. Follow with your head. Repeat with the other arm.

⇨ Kneel on all fours, hands under your shoulders, dig your toes into the ground and inhale. Exhale as you move your hips into the air, straightening your legs. Inhale to draw your knees towards your thighs and exhale as you push your hips to the ground. Inhale and draw your shoulders away from your ears, then exhale as you push your heels to the ground, and hold the position for 5–10 breaths.

⇨ Inhale as you move your hips towards the ground, drawing your shoulders away from your ears, and looking up. Then exhale as you arch like a cat, looking down at your navel. Inhale to return to your knees then take your buttocks back to your heels.

⇨ Stand upright, draw your knees up towards your thighs, lengthen your neck and inhale. Then exhale as you jump wide, taking your arms out in line with the top of your shoulders, then inhale. As you exhale, turn your head to look over your left fingers, inhale, then exhale as your left leg bends forward, making sure not to take your knee beyond 90 degrees. Hold the position for 10 breaths, keeping your shoulders away from your ears and making sure not to strain. Inhale to return to centre, then repeat to bend the right leg.

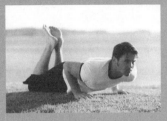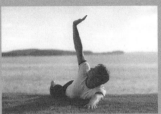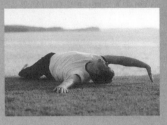

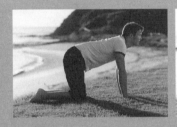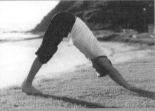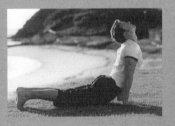

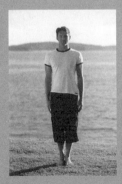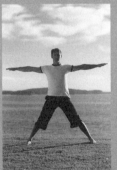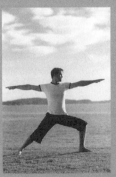

LATE SUMMER CLASS (SPLEEN AND STOMACH ENERGY)

⇨ Lie on your back, your knees bent, your feet hip width apart and close to your buttocks. Hold onto your ankles or press your palms into the ground. Inhale to prepare. As you exhale, take your left knee down towards your right foot, keeping your right leg vertical. Inhale to return to centre. Repeat on the other side. Repeat both sides 10 times.

⇨ Lie on your back, your knees bent, your feet hip width apart and close to your buttocks. Your arms should be extended, and palms pressed into the ground. Inhale to prepare. Then as you exhale, lift your hips up and away from the floor, using your palms, until your hips are in line with your chest. Inhale to return slowly to the ground. Repeat 5–10 times.

⇨ Lift your hips as in the above position, hold and inhale, then as you exhale, slide your left leg on the ground, pointing your toes. Inhale, and exhale to slowly lift your leg into a vertical position, pointing your toes, keeping the hips lifted off the ground. Inhale to slowly lower your leg. Repeat 10 times, rest, then repeat with the other leg.

⇨ Lie on your back, bend your knees out and push the soles of your feet together. They should be in line with your navel, where the calves would normally be. Place your palms below your navel, and inhale to prepare. As you exhale, slowly curl up through the upper body, sliding your hands towards your throat. Inhale to slowly curl down, taking your hands back down to the navel. Repeat 10 times.

⇨ Lie on your back, your legs extended and toes pulled back. Place your elbows close to your sides, hands in fists. Inhale to prepare. As you exhale, push up through your elbows to lift only the chest, making sure not to strain or push through the neck. Inhale to return to the ground, and exhale to repeat the lift. Repeat 5 times.

⇨ Lie on your back, inhale and exhale as you bend your knees to your chest, then extend the legs vertically above your hips. Inhale, then exhale as you curl up with the torso, arms extended, as you take your fingers close to your extended toes. Hold the position for three breaths. Repeat 5 times.

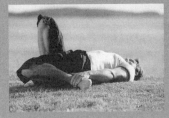
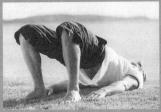
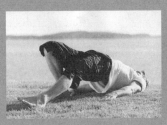

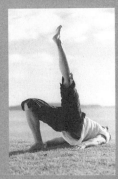
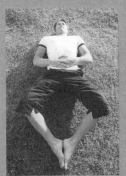

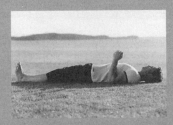
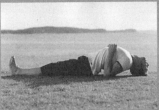
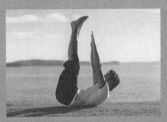

⇨ Lie on your belly, arms and legs extended. Inhale to prepare. Exhale as you lift your arms and legs off the ground. Your neck should remain aligned with your spine and not strained. Inhale to slowly return to the ground. Repeat 10 times.

⇨ Lie on your belly, place your heels on your buttocks and hold the tops of your feet or ankles. Inhale to prepare. As you exhale, lift your torso and knees off the ground, using your arms and legs. You should not strain your neck. Inhale to return to the ground. Repeat 5 times.

⇨ Kneel and rest your buttocks on your heels. Look forward and inhale. Exhale as you come forward through with the chest and inhale as you straighten your arms and look above, drawing your shoulders away from your ears. Exhale as you arch like a cat, looking at your navel. Inhale as you take your buttocks back to your heels, looking forward. Repeat the sequence twice.

⇨ Lie on your back, press your palms together and the soles of your feet together, knees and elbows are wide. Inhale to prepare and exhale as you extend your hands over your head and slide your legs along the ground (only as far as you can without taking the soles of your feet apart). Inhale to return to centre. Repeat with your feet just above the ground, but if it's too difficult, slide them along the ground. Repeat 5–10 times.

⇨ Lie on your back, interlock your fingers in front of your knees. Inhale to prepare. Exhale as you curl your head towards your knees, bringing your knees towards your chest. Inhale then exhale to return to the ground. Repeat 5 times.

⇨ Rest pose: Lie on your back, legs and arms extended, palms facing up, feet flopped out to the sides.

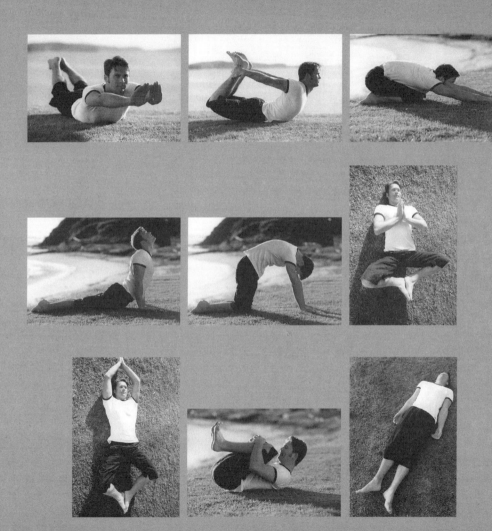

AUTUMN CLASS (LUNGS AND LARGE INTESTINE ENERGY)

⇨ Sit, kneeling, and tuck your thumbs into fists. Take in a big breath, hold it, and lightly pound the top of your chest. When you can't hold your breath any more, exhale as you take your upper body forward until your forehead touches the ground (pose of child), your fists close to your sides.

⇨ Sit, kneeling, and tuck your thumbs into fists. Inhale as you raise your arms above your head, hold your breath and pump your fists into the air 20 times. When you can't hold your breath any more, exhale as you go into pose of child.

⇨ Sit, kneeling, and tuck your thumbs into fists. Inhale as you raise your arms above your head, hold your breath, then lightly pound the lower area and sides of your chest. When you can't hold your breath any more, exhale and go into pose of child.

⇨ Sit with your legs straight, bring your right foot to rest just above the left knee and let it flop. Extend your arms to the front, pulling your shoulders away from your ears. Pull back the toes of both feet, and inhale as you lift out of your chest. Exhale as you lean forward, keeping your toes pulled back. Inhale to return to centre. Exhale as you lean halfway back, then inhale to return to centre. Repeat 10 times on each side.

⇨ Lie on your back, resting your left foot over your right knee. Hold onto your shin and knee and inhale to prepare. Exhale as you pull your knee towards your chest, curling your head towards your knee. Inhale to return to the ground. Repeat for 5 breaths each side.

⇨ Lie on your back with your feet together, toes pulled back, arms out at 90 degrees, palms pressed into the ground. Inhale to prepare, then exhale as you lift your right leg vertically, keeping your toes pulled back. Inhale, then exhale as you take your right leg over to the left side of your body, towards the ground, turning your head to look towards the right hand. Inhale to take your leg back to vertical, then exhale as you take your leg to the right side, looking towards your left hand. Repeat 5–10 times then repeat on the left leg.

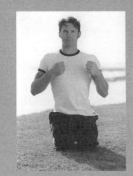
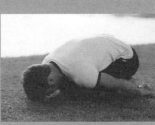
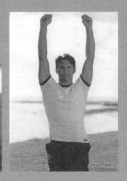

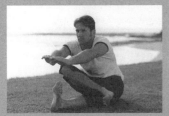
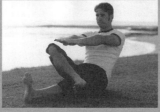
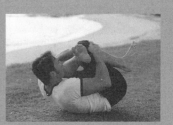

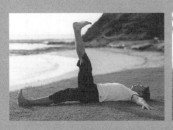
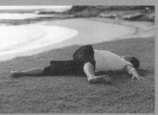
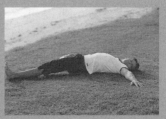

⇨ Lie on your back, hands in fists, arms bent in strong-arm position, turn in toes, heels out, ground your back into the ground and inhale. Exhale as you lift your legs 15 cm, keeping your toes together and your lower back on the ground. If this is too difficult, try only one leg. Repeat 5–10 times.

⇨ Lying in the above position, legs wider than hips, inhale and exhale as you lift your legs 15 cm, keeping the toes together and lower back on the ground. If too difficult, lift only one leg. Repeat 5–10 times.

⇨ Lying in the above position, with legs as wide as possible, inhale then exhale as you lift your legs 15 cm, keeping your toes together and lower back on the ground. If too difficult lift only one leg. Repeat 5–10 times.

⇨ Lying on your back, feet together, bring feet close to your buttocks, drop your knees to the right, push your right thumb into the space between your left thumb and forefinger, rest your hands on your hips, and inhale. Exhale as you slowly curl up while pushing the point on your hand, inhale to return slowly down, keeping the tension on the belly. Repeat 8–10 times; repeat on the other side.

⇨ Lie on the ground, interlock your fingers behind your head, legs extended, toes pulled back, inhale. Exhale as you curl your head up, keeping your elbows on the ground. Inhale to return slowly down. Repeat 5 times.

⇨ Inhale, then exhale as you curl your head up and squeeze your elbows together. Inhale and return slowly down, opening your elbows. Repeat 5 times.

⇨ Lie on your belly, hands close to your chest, fingers pointing towards your feet (or out to the side if too difficult), inhale. Squeeze your elbows together as you exhale and try to come halfway up in a push-up. Inhale and return back down. Repeat 5 times. Inhale, then exhale as you squeeze your elbows together and push up. Hold and inhale, rock forwards and backwards, exhaling until out of breath, and try to rock a few more times. Collapse and rest.

⇨ Sit with buttocks to heels, looking forward, inhale. Exhale as you come forward through with the chest and inhale as you straighten your arms and look above, drawing your shoulders away from your ears. Exhale as you arch like a cat, looking at your navel. Inhale as you take your buttocks to your heels, looking forward. Repeat sequence twice.

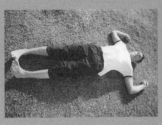
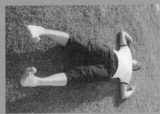
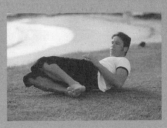

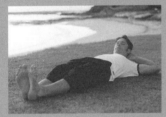
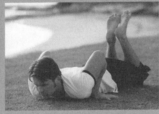
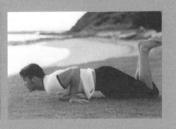

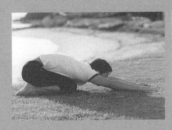
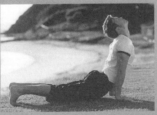
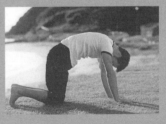

WINTER CLASS (KIDNEYS AND BLADDER ENERGY)

⇨ Sit with legs in front, toes pulled back, inhale to lift out of your chest, then exhale as you move forward and hold the back of your calves or feet. Inhale, then exhale as you lean forward, taking your chest towards your knees, keeping your shoulders away from your knees. Do not strain, hold for 5 breaths.

⇨ Sit with legs in front, place the sole of your right foot along the left calf muscle, inhale to lift out of your chest, arms forward. Exhale as you move forward, keeping your toes pulled back. Inhale and return to centre. Exhale to lean halfway back, then inhale to return to centre. Repeat the sequence 5 times.

⇨ Lie on your back with your feet close to your buttocks hip width apart. Hold onto your ankles or push your palms into the ground, inhale. Exhale as you push your hips up into the air, squeezing your buttocks. Inhale and return slowly down. Repeat 5 times.

⇨ Lying in the above position, inhale then exhale as you push your hips up into the air, squeezing your buttocks. Hold the position for 5 breaths, inhale, then exhale as you take your hips over to the right (small movement). Inhale and return to centre, exhale as you take your hips to the left. Repeat 5 times.

⇨ Lie on your back, knees lifted, interlock your fingers and place hands behind your head. Place feet wider than hips, with feet as far away from your body as possible without your soles coming off the ground. Inhale to prepare. Exhale as you slowly curl up, twisting your right elbow towards your left knee. Inhale to twist back to centre and curl back down to the ground. Repeat 5 times on each side.

⇨ Lie on your back with the soles of your feet together, close to your buttocks, knees wide and hands on hips, inhale. Exhale as you curl up slowly, inhale and slowly return down, keeping the tension in your belly. Repeat 5 times.

⇨ Lie on your belly, arms outstretched, inhale. Exhale as you lift your left arm and right leg into the air. Inhale and bring your limbs down. Repeat, alternating sides, 10 times.

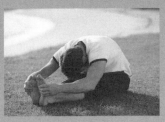 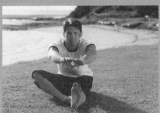 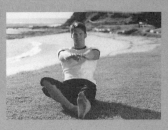

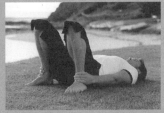 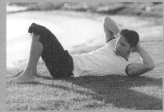 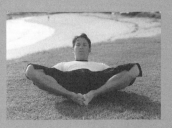

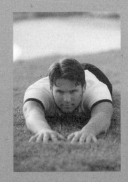 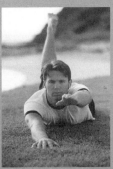

⇨ Lie on your belly, arms outstretched, inhale, then exhale to lift your left arm and left leg into the air. Inhale and bring limbs down. Repeat, alternating sides, 10 times.

⇨ Lie on your belly, take your arms and legs as wide as possible, inhale, then exhale as you lift your limbs into the air. Flex your toes towards the ground and fingers upwards, hold, inhale, then exhale as you bring your arms and legs together. Inhale to open limbs wide and repeat 5 times. Collapse and rest.

⇨ Lie on your belly, with your knees wide, soles of your feet together and hands by chest. Inhale, then exhale as you lift your torso and hands off the ground. Inhale, holding them up, then exhale as you bend around to the right side, keeping your elbows pulled back. Inhale to return to centre, exhale and repeat on the other side. Repeat both sides 10 times. (This position is for sexual energy.)

⇨ Rest on all fours, with hands under your shoulders, inhale, then exhale to arch like a cat, looking towards your navel. Inhale and return to centre, then exhale as you sag like a cow, looking up to the sky. Inhale and return to centre. Repeat the sequence 5 times.

⇨ Sit with your buttocks to your heels, looking forward. Inhale, then exhale as you come forward with the chest. Inhale as you straighten your arms and look above, drawing your shoulders away from your ears. Exhale as you arch like a cat, looking at your navel. Inhale as you take your buttocks back to your heels, looking forward. Repeat the sequence twice.

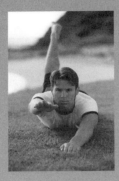
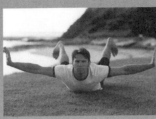
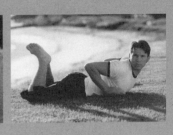

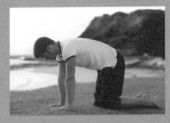
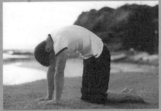
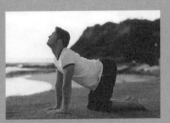

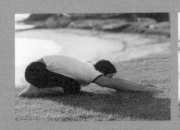
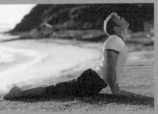
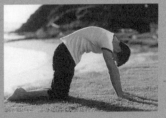

BACK CLASS

⇨ Lie on your belly, arms outstretched, inhale. Exhale as you lift your left arm and your right leg into the air. Inhale and lower your limbs down. Repeat 10 times, alternating on each side.

⇨ Lie on your belly, inhale and exhale lifting your left arm and left leg up into the air. Inhale to lower your limbs. Repeat alternating sides 10 times.

⇨ Lie on your belly, take your arms and legs as wide as possible, inhale. Exhale as you lift your limbs into the air, flexing your toes towards the ground and your fingers upwards. Hold the pose, inhale, then exhale bringing your limbs together. Inhale to open limbs wide and repeat 5 times. Collapse and rest.

⇨ Lie on your belly with your knees wide, soles of your feet together, hands by chest, and inhale. Exhale as you lift your torso and hands off the ground. Inhale holding them up, exhale bending around to the right side, keeping your elbows pulled back. Inhale to return to centre, exhale and repeat on the other side. Repeat both sides 10 times.

⇨ Lie on your belly with your legs just wider than hip width, toes dug into the ground, right arm out to the side and left hand over your head. Inhale, then exhale as you take your right arm into a vertical position, keeping your knees on the ground. Flex your hand and stretch through the middle finger as you try to take it to the ground. Inhale and bring down your arm. Repeat 5 times. Inhale, then exhale as you lift your arm out as far as possible, keeping your knees on the ground, then follow with your head. Hold for 3–5 breaths.

⇨ Kneel on all fours, with your hands under your shoulders, dig your toes into the ground and inhale. Exhale as you move your hips up into the air, straightening your legs. Inhale drawing your knees into your thighs and exhale as you push your elbows to the ground. Inhale drawing your shoulders away from your ears, then exhale as you push your heels to the ground, and hold for 5–10 breaths.

Inhale as you move your hips towards the ground, drawing your shoulders away from your ears, looking above. Exhale as you arch like a cat, looking at your navel. Inhale taking your buttocks back to your heels.

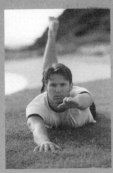
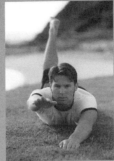
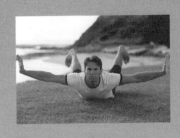

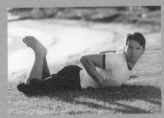
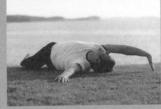
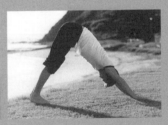

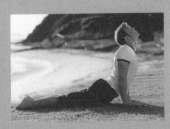
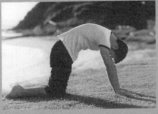
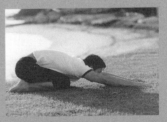

⇨ Lie on your back, interlock your fingers and place your hands behind your head. Place your feet wider than your hips with your feet as far away from the body as possible, without your soles coming off the ground, inhale. Exhale as you slowly curl up, and twist your right elbow towards your left knee, then inhale slowly twisting towards the centre, then curling down to the ground. Repeat 5 times, holding the curl for 3 breaths each time.

⇨ Lie on your back, legs extended, toes pulled back, hands in fists, elbows close to your chest, and inhale. Exhale pushing up only your chest, inhale and return down. If there's no pressure on your neck, exhale and push your chest up and come onto the top of your head, pushing through your elbows at all times. Inhale and return slowly down.

⇨ Lie on your back, interlock your fingers in front of your left knee and inhale. Exhale curling up, pushing your knee away and using it to help you come all the way up. Repeat on the other side.

⇨ Lie on the ground with your feet together, toes pulled back, arms out at 90 degrees and your palms into the ground, inhale. Exhale as you lift your right leg up into a vertical position, keeping your toes pulled back. Inhale, then exhale as you take your right leg over to the left side, looking towards your right hand. Inhale as you take your leg back into vertical, then exhale as your leg goes down to the right side, looking towards your left hand. Repeat with the other leg.

⇨ Lie on your back, interlock your fingers in front of your knees, inhale. Exhale as you curl your head towards your knees and bring your knees towards your chest. Repeat 5 times.

⇨ Lie on your back, legs extended, your right arm at a right angle to your torso, palm facing down. Inhale and bring your right foot up next to your left knee. Exhale as you take your right knee down to the left, looking towards your right hand. Hold the pose for 5–10 breaths. Repeat on the other side.

⇨ Rest pose: Lie on your back, palms up, legs extended, feet flopped out.

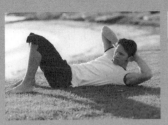 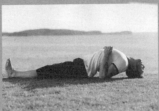 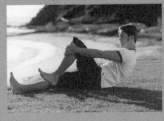

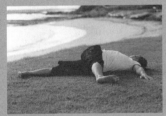 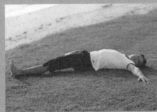 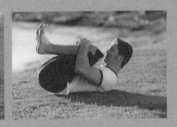

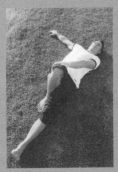 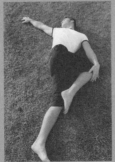 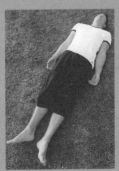

CHAPTER 7

MASSAGE

Pain and stiffness in the body are usually signs that something is wrong. Avoiding to address these just compounds the problem. Self-massage therapy is something we can all do, and no matter how little effect you think you are having when self massaging, you will be healing yourself. In this chapter you will find quick ways to release tension and tips on how to revitalise yourself.

Before attempting any massage, please check with your doctor if you suffer any bone or muscular conditions, bruise easily or have haemophilia.

What is massage

We all have a natural connection with our bodies, yet we tend to ignore what we already know. For example, if someone complains of a headache, they instinctively take their hand to their head and squeeze for a moment. Massage helps to release stress and relieve muscle pain, headache, nausea and fatigue.

In oriental medical philosophy, it is said that, 'Where there is pain there is blockage'. The purpose of massage, shiatsu and acupuncture is to remove the blockages of chi (energy) and blood flow circulation. By restoring the circulation of chi and blood through the body, you can eliminate pain. A dull ache is a sign that chi is stagnant. A sharp pain indicates blood stagnation.

You need to choose the right type of massage for the pain or tension you feel. When stiffness or pain diminishes with pressure applied, it is called tonifying. When the pain increases with pressure, you are sedating the area. You can work above and below this area to sedate the area without hurting yourself. You can pick a specific point to work on or you can give yourself a general self-massage.

At the end of the day, there really are no right or wrong techniques. You will find that you only use what works for you.

Pressure point technique

Apply bearable pressure on the area with the bulbs of the fingers and thumbs for at least three seconds, pause then continue. I generally count internally 1000, 2000,

3000, pause, release, then repeat. You can substitute this with any technique that comes to mind, such as sliding the thumb over the point, using your palms or whatever works best for you. Be very gentle with any pressure around the face.

ACCURACY

It does not matter if you feel you are not pressing on an exact pressure point, with time and experience you shall soon discover that you have a natural affinity with finding where the tension lies. The more you try, the better you will get at it. I believe we have an inherent connection with our own bodies, yet, commonly, this trust and knowledge in one's own capabilities is ignored and even temporarily discarded.

GETTING STARTED

See if some of the following points bring about a change in how you feel. First, take a mental snapshot of how your body feels—what feels tight, sore, heavy, light. Apply pressure only to a level that is comfortable to you. Do not bring yourself to the point of tears! Surrender and allow the tension to release. All the experiences and situations in your life have created this build-up of tension in your body—now is your opportunity to release it. Allow it to happen.

SELF-MASSAGE ROUTINE

Work through the whole body or simply target where most of your tension is.

SHOULDERS

Take your right hand and rest it on the top of your left shoulder. Slowly press down with the fingers. What amount of pressure feels okay for you? Is your shoulder sore/tense? Become aware of the tension. Move your fingers forwards and backwards along the shoulder, pushing down, trying to find the spot that is the most uncomfortable. When you have found the spot, take a big breath and gently breathe out as you apply pressure. Relax the pressure, breathe and repeat the step twice more. How does that shoulder feel now? Move on to the right shoulder, repeat the massage and compare it with your left shoulder.

Take notice of how quickly some pressure can cause a shift of awareness in the body and most importantly the release of tension within the body. What else has shifted—has your posture altered, or is your breath deeper and fuller? Enjoy this experience.

HEAD

Start at the base of the skull. Place both hands behind your head and use the first two fingers on both hands to *gently* push upwards into the base of the skull. If you feel like you need more pressure, you can use your thumbs instead. Hold the pressure for around three seconds, pause, then release. Then repeat twice.

From this point, you can move your hands further apart, about two fingerwidths. Gently push the fingers up into the base of the skull again and repeat the steps and pressure techniques you have been using already. Continue moving your fingers further apart, applying pressure at each point, until you have worked your way to near your ears.

Now it's time to work from the top of the skull. Take both hands and spread them over the top of your head, with the first three fingers touching each other. Gently push down onto the skull and hold for a count of three, pause, then release. Move your hands about two fingerwidths apart and reapply the pressure as before. Slide your fingers further from the centre and repeat.

Don't worry about hitting the exact area, try moving the hands around to see what works for you. Remember what it's like when you get a shampoo at the hairdresser—it's very relaxing and enjoyable regardless of what techniques they use. Massage is like that, it all works in one way or another!

FACE

The face is a delicate area, so don't apply so much pressure that you end up with black eyes. You can still use very gentle pressure for great results. Apply the pressure at each step, hold for a count of three, pause, release, then repeat each step twice.

Place your fingers on the centre of your forehead with the palms facing down and apply pressure to the forehead. Then slide your hands towards the side of your face until the fingertips are in line with the centre of your eyebrows and apply pressure. Slide your hands and fingers outwards once more until they line up with the outside edge of your eyebrows and apply pressure. Take each thumb to the centre of each eyebrow and push up gently into the depression.

Use a lighter pressure on and around the eyes. Close your eyelids. Place the first three fingers of each hand on the eyelids and push up gently to the top side of the eye sockets. Then gently apply pressure to the eye. Slide the fingers down and gently push onto the bottom of the eye socket.

Place the tip of your second finger over the first fingertip to increase the pressure. Place the 'double fingers' onto either side of your nose near the top before the nose cartilage begins, where your nose and cheek meet. Gently apply pressure to the edge. Slide the 'double fingers' halfway towards the bottom of your nose, and gently push into the edge of your nose. Slide the 'double fingers' down to the outside edge of the nostril flare and gently apply pressure.

Place your two fingers side by side and gently apply pressure to the cheek bones near your nose. Move fingers to the centre of your cheek bones, you should find a small depression at this point, and gently apply pressure. Slide your fingers to the outside edge of your cheek bones and apply pressure.

Place your two fingers, side by side on your temples and gently apply pressure.

With 'double fingers' gently press beneath the centre of your nose, above the top of your lips. Place the 'double fingers' onto the outside corner of your lips and apply pressure. Place 'double fingers' beneath the centre of your bottom lip and apply pressure.

Using your thumbs, push upwards underneath your chin.

THROAT

Use only light pressure in this area. As above, apply pressure at each point for a count of three, pause and release, then repeat twice.

Place two fingers, side by side, on either side of the windpipe and gently push down. Slide your fingers down to the middle of the throat, on either side of the windpipe, and apply pressure. Move to the bottom of the throat and apply pressure.

Slide your fingers a little further away from the centre of the throat and work down as before, applying pressure at the top, middle and bottom of the throat.

Take your fingers even further outwards and repeat the pressure at the top, middle and bottom.

NECK

Working with two fingers side by side, apply pressure on either side of the centre of the neck at the top. Work down the neck in this manner, applying pressure at the middle and then the bottom. Now move your fingers about two fingerwidths away from the centre, and apply pressure at the three points, top, middle and bottom, down towards the shoulders. Finally, move your fingers in line with the edge of the base of the skull and work down to the bottom in a straight line as before.

HANDS

The beauty of the hands is that we can massage them without anyone else really knowing—for example, you can work these points while waiting in a queue.

Start by taking the right thumb and place it over the top of the space between the left thumb and forefinger. Push down, gently squeeze both the thumb and forefinger together, hold for three seconds, pause and release, then repeat twice. Slide the thumb down into the middle of this 'webbed' area and gently apply pressure by squeezing. Finally, slide the thumb down to the edge of the 'webbing' and apply pressure. If it makes it easier to identify these points, think of the first point as the mountain, the second as the valley and the last as the gorge.

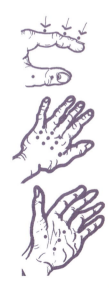

Continue and work on to the space in between the first and second finger then repeat the process with the other two finger junctions.

Next, move on to the fingers. Basically there are three points on the fingers, the only exception being the thumb where there are two. Start with the first finger, the first point is below the knuckle, near the hand. Push down with the thumb and squeeze with the forefinger at the same time. Then slide the thumb down to between the two knuckles and apply pressure. Slide the thumb and forefinger down to squeeze the base of the thumbnail. Work each finger and the thumb, then work the sides of the fingers and thumbs in the same manner.

To work the palm of the hand, push with the thumb and gently squeeze on the back of the hand at the same time. Apply pressure as shown in the illustrations.

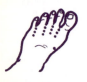

Feet
The feet are similar to our hands, so we can work them in pretty much the same manner. Have a look at these illustrations if you are not sure. Improvise and knead into the sole of the foot more than you did the palms. Just have fun, and give your feet the treat they deserve—think of how many kilometres they have taken you.

Remember, massage can be as short or as long as you want. You can use it on the way to or from work. You can use it while working at the computer, or even before going to bed. We have only brushed on the surface of massage techniques but even with these simple techniques you can get instant benefits.

22 MAJOR PRESSURE POINTS IN THE BODY

1. Pericardium—PC 6
   Two thumbwidths up from the wrists.
   Nausea, unsettled emotions affecting our digestion, insomnia.

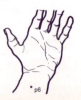

p6

2. Colon—LI 4
   Beginning of colds and flus, headaches, toothaches, problems
   with the head, stimulates intestinal function, use locally for
   hand problems.

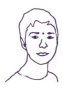

3. Yin Tang
   Point between eyebrows higher than the nose bridge.
   Headaches, insomnia, tension headaches, good for busy minds,
   sinus problems, calms and sedates.

4. Governor vessel 20
   Find the tip of the ears, then draw a line up until the fingers
   meet at the top of the head.
   Calming, insomnia, stimulating brain function, headaches at
   the top of the head, haemorrhoids.

5. Gall bladder—GB21
   Highest point on the shoulder muscle.
   Tight shoulder tension, releasing knots and
   stops shooting pain up from shoulder to skull.

6. Gall bladder—GB 20 GB 12 BL 10 Occiputs
   Great for releasing neck tension.

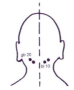

7. Heart—HT 7
   Next to pisiform on top of wrist (inside of bump).
   Upset emotions, shock, grieving, stress.

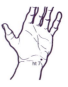

8. Colon—LI 11
   End of elbow crease when the arm is flexed.
   Constipation, diarrhoea.

9. Conception vessel—CV 17 Ren Mei
   In line with nipples, or fourth intercostal.
   Closed tight chest, grief, asthmatics.

10. Conception vessel—CV 12
    Four thumbwidths above the belly button, in line with centre of body.
    Digestion problems—reflux, excessive eating, bloating, diarrhoea.

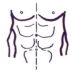

11. Stomach—ST 30
    Top of pubic bone, both sides.
    Period pain, irregular menstruation, impotence, swollen testicles and penis.

WARNING: Do not do pressure points 11 or 15 if pregnant!

12. Stomach—ST 36 Three mile legs
    Three thumbwidths beneath the outside knee eye (bottom of the
    knee)—fingerwidth away from the shinbone.
    Extra energy, stimulates digestive function, revives consciousness,
    diarrhoea, vomiting and belching.

13. Gall bladder—GB 34
    Fibia.
    Muscle tension, cramps, spasms, ligament or tendon damage, or even just after
    a hard work-out.

14. Bladder—BL 40
    Centre of the back of the knee crease.
    Acute and chronic lumbar pain, back of knee problems,
    hamstring tightness.

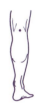

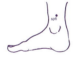

15. Spleen—SP 6
    Three thumbwidths up from top of inside ankle bone.
    Ankle problems, period pain, late menstruation, swollen ankles.

16. Liver—LV 3
    In between the big toe and second toe metatarsals.
    Headaches, stressed out, sore eyes, irritable behaviour,
    snappy, angry, bad-tempered emotions.

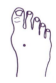

17. Kidneys—KI 1
    Sore feet, grounding when feeling disconnected.

18. Kidneys—KI 3

   Ankle bone, between Achilles tendon and the peak of the ankle bone.
   Urinary functions, black under eyes, boosting energy levels.

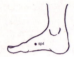

19. Spleen—SP 4

   Just in front of the bump on the arch of the foot.
   Digestion, depression, insomnia, pain in feet.

20. Liver—LI 20

   Outside of nostril flares.
   Sinus.

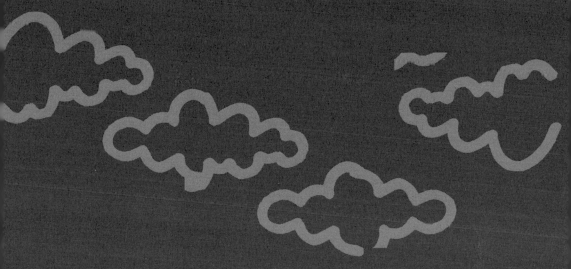

PART III

THE SPIRIT

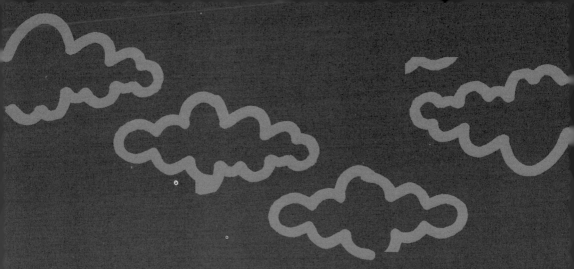

CHAPTER 8

THE REAL YOU

This chapter is about revealing to yourself who you really are, and how we all can fall into routines that mean we spend a large portion of our lives being someone we don't want to be, and doing things we don't want to do.

Everyone has beliefs about the world and themselves which influence the way they live their lives. These beliefs create patterns of behaviour. There are various personal development programs and psychological schools of thought that can help to identify those beliefs and patterns. The principles used in this chapter are based upon the ones that have worked for me. With respect to my beliefs, I acknowledge my greatest mentor is Darren Ward who imparted his wisdom to me through his course Living from Greatness.

FEELING WHOLE

Sometime in the past, you made an assumption that something was missing in your life. You have since spent most of your time looking for it, trying to make amends for something you think you did not receive. The reality is, you are already complete.

The realisation that you are already complete doesn't mean you give up any quest—be it religion, the clothes you wear or the people you see. It just involves you being brave enough to reveal your true self to yourself and others. People can spend their whole lives searching for something they already possess—their real (complete) self, when all they needed to do is to reveal it.

We are brought up in various cultures, with different values, languages and spiritual and religious beliefs. No matter where you go, everyone has a philosophy about why and what we are here for. But rarely do we feel content with these notions.

We all have a burning desire to find out more about ourselves, and what is special about us. Although we can go to extraordinary lengths to look, act and be like others, we are all unique and amazing! At the end of the day, it doesn't matter where you were born, what culture you were brought up in, who your parents are, or what you have or have not done with your life. Why? Because you are already complete. It's just that you made an assumption very early in your life that something was missing, and have spent the rest of your life making this perceived thing that you feel is missing a part of yourself—making it come true.

To fully appreciate what this means, you need to recognise some key premises. A premise is just an idea or assumption that may be right or it may be wrong.

Below are the premises which I think underline our need for validation and ways to counteract the premise to get what we want from life. You do not have to believe in the premises to begin with, but you may change your tune as you read on. For now, try to stay open-minded and work out whether, or how much, these premises ring true to you.

PREMISES

YOU SEEK VALIDATION FROM YOUR PARENTS

We all try to seek one hundred per cent validation from our parents, whether they are alive and known to us or are no longer a part of our lives. In truth, we can never receive this kind of validation from anyone, so we end up with a wound deep inside our inner self.

At some time in our early childhood, which we may or may not remember, we have all encountered a situation where we did not get complete validation of our parents' love for us. It could have been something quite ordinary, such as a parent telling their child that they have been naughty and sending them off to bed. From a child's point of view, what their parent has done is show the child that they do not love them one hundred per cent. Whether the parent loves them that much or not is irrelevant. If it becomes true in the mind of the child, for the rest of that child's life, they carry a wound based on the belief that they did not receive the validation they required. They then spend their life creating beliefs and forming strategies in their personalities to gain this validation.

This is a very important premise. It can be hard to accept. Try to be open-minded and give yourself some time to digest it. Think about times in your childhood and later when someone disappointed you greatly. Ask yourself if what you were asking from that person was reasonable.

YOU CREATE BELIEFS ABOUT YOURSELF AND THE WORLD

From our disappointments and lack of validation from others, we make assumptions, create beliefs and start to establish patterns that stay with us for the rest of our lives. This may simply be the belief that we are not good enough, or not lovable. There are many beliefs which we may play out for the rest of our lives to compensate for not receiving complete validation from our parents. This means that a lot of the things you are doing and the way you see the world is directly caused by these beliefs.

If you take the time to look at yourself in the broader context of how your upbringing has affected your life, you can start to understand how a particular wound moulded your beliefs.

YOU CREATE STRATEGIES/PERSONALITIES

From our beliefs we create the life we live today. Our beliefs about ourselves are correct. If you have the belief that you are not good enough, you could spend your whole life trying to be good enough. So you might be an over-achiever—perhaps you attain lots of academic qualifications, through your hard work and success, but you often burn out in the process. The strategy you develop to compensate for not feeling good enough is to over-achieve, which does not resolve your belief.

Our beliefs can control our lives. *Living from Greatness* tells us that some of the major beliefs and strategies that people follow include:

I'm unworthy	Will try to seek love and approval, take the steps to attract it, but often reject it.
I'm not good enough	Strives to achieve completion through working hard and creating success, often burning out in the process.
I don't belong	Will try to become part of a group and have a place where they belong in order to find out who they are.

I need to control myself	Will try to control themselves and others, and will generally follow rules to make up for the lack of orientation in their life.
I can't trust myself, others or the world	Will try to do things on their own or, when working with others, will test them by demanding guarantees to plan a safe road for survival.
I don't have the capacity	Will pretend they don't have the resource or time to get things done and will either over-commit or under-commit themselves to tasks at hand.
I'm insignificant	Will detach themselves from things and not ask for what they really want to ensure they avoid any conflict.
There is a right way	Will do things according to certain methods and systems, using a rigid approach to reaffirm their belief that there is always a right way, one they can predict.
There is a way things are	Will seek lots of knowledge so that they can be certain they know what to do with everything.
I'm powerless	Will set up power bases to appear powerful, will act power hungry or as a victim of being powerless.
I'm not allowed to be capable	Will under-achieve rather than over-achieve and avoid situations where they will test their capabilities, although they are really seeking the freedom they can get from doing what they really want.
I need to be perfect	Will never begin what they want and destroy what they have created so that they will not be found out to be imperfect. They believe that perfection exists and it's something one needs to be. They seek to find peace and resolve their life.

Do any of these beliefs and strategies seem familiar?

YOU PERPETUATE THE REALITY YOU CREATED UNLESS . . .

If you do not become aware of your wounds and beliefs, you will continue to live trying to seek that one hundred per cent validation. You will keep living your life feeling unsatisfied, discontent and searching for meaning when you already have the answer within you.

YOU ARE ALREADY COMPLETE

The only real problems you have are those that you create through your own ego and from the beliefs and strategies you created from it. Love, peace and happiness are all inside you. It cannot be given to you, it must come from within, by understanding the truth about yourself and how you live your life. If you are aware of what is really going on, you live the truth and will embrace your real self and greatness.

If I become a more peaceful, happy and loving person, would the world change? I would hope so. Why? If I change then the world around me changes. I accept people as they are and do not try to change them. The onus to change my world then does not fall on others but on me alone. Think about how much conflict would dissipate if we all realised that what we are searching for lies within. Our lives would be full of joy and fun if we were all doing what we love.

What about my neighbour, who I can't stand, or my tyrannic boss? How often do we want to change other people—'If only that person would . . .' or 'I wish they would realise . . .'? If the person does not change, then the person who wants them to change feels frustrated and never escapes the wrath of discontentment because they are looking outside for the solution. We can only change ourselves, not others.

Everyone, including you, has the capacity to change, but if you close yourself off to awareness then you will never know what you possess. You will be destined to spend your whole life doing all sorts of activities trying to find what you already have within you—completion, love, peace and happiness.

Make this your mantra: I am already complete.

YOU CAN CREATE THE LIFE YOU WANT

We all create and receive every day. The point we are aiming for is a place where we can accept what we create and receive. The two go hand in hand. This means you have to be open to both engaging yourself to create change and then receiving what you have created.

Think about how many of us work tirelessly to achieve tasks yet never choose to receive any recognition or become aware of the journey we have undertaken. This thought may be the springboard for you to create change and receive its rewards—you can do it.

EMBRACING YOUR WOUNDS

Rather than running around for the rest of your life trying to achieve validation from your parents, acknowledge that it is irrelevant. If you embrace what you have been working so hard to avoid, your wound, you will be filled with a sense of contentment and happiness. This is not always easy because we all spend our whole lives avoiding and covering up our wounds. We might be successful but it may not be the life we truly want to live.

YOUR DARK SIDE

The 'dark side' is what we fear the most in ourselves, that fear which creates our wounds. When we drop all our pretences, then our true self remains. By embracing our wounds, our dark side, we embrace our real selves.

Imagine a successful stockbroker who would love to be a teacher. Although he may be great at what he does, there is something else that he would rather be. He is not going to be entirely happy, or of real service to the people in his lives, until he accepts that what he would love to do is a worthwhile choice, until he embraces his fear, his dark side.

I always believed I had to study more, to do another course, to be better. After university I'd start another course, satisfying my ego but taking me further away from what I really wanted to do.

Although some of the decisions that our ego makes seem very reasonable, they can be completely off course. You need to separate what you want and what your ego wants.

YOUR EGO VERSUS YOUR WANTS

Do you ever feel that you would like to do things but something inside you says no? Or perhaps you started to do something you always wanted to do only to be let down by your own doubts, concerns and worries. It can be frustrating when you start trying to work out what's not working in your life! You may be successful in your career, relationships and family, yet something is still missing. The problem is that our real self wants to do what it really loves but our ego stops us by telling us things like: 'Don't be silly, you don't want to give away your career to do that!'

Right now my ego wants to go surfing, swim and play, which is part of my strategy—to fill up my time with never-ending activities that are fun but take me away from what I really want to do, which, at the moment, is to finish this book. Don't get me wrong, a lot of the time I will play, but I try to do it only when I really want to do it, not just for the sake of it.

There's nothing wrong with dividing your attention between other activities if that's what you really want to do. For me, not working on my book will perpetuate my reality of not completing projects, or starting with good ideas and not finishing them so I cannot succeed and receive the rewards of completing them. There are lots of beliefs that come into play, but, at the end of the day, I just have to ask myself, what would I really love to do? Is it to be of service to others by shining the light of truth into their lives, or is it to procrastinate through surfing, when the waves aren't that good anyway!

When we go for what we love, for what we want to do, things start to happen in ways that defy logic, our rational mind. We start to believe and trust in our intuition and our ability to create what we really love.

YOUR INTUITION

Intuition is not our rational thought but our instinct and higher self which works effortlessly. We all know the feeling we get in the stomach when something is not quite right and when it is. This is a part of our intuition. The more you can use it, the more you will be operating from your real self rather than from your head, your beliefs, your wound, patterns and, of course, your ego!

When you use your intuition, you operate from the right side of the brain. Information is processed in a wholistic manner that involves mental imagery, feelings and insights. This is a completely different approach to using the left side of the brain, which uses logical, rational and linear thought processes. We tend to fall into the trap of following the rational left side, which keeps us more aligned with following the beliefs and patterns we have established in our lives.

When we get in touch with our intuition, we free our minds of these bonds and can be open to receiving insights and direction aligned with our true selves.

EXERCISES—FINDING THE REAL YOU

To do these exercises all you need is a comfy chair in a quiet place where you will not be disturbed and a pen and note pad so you can start writing as soon as you have finished the visualisation. When writing about your image, if at any time you feel stuck, just keep writing. You will still be connecting with your inner self through your stream of consciousness.

Before each visualisation, close your eyes and take a big breath into your belly, then let the breath out with a big 'Aaaarggghhh'. Take in a bigger breath, then let the breath go completely. Acknowledge any thoughts or feelings you have, but don't be concerned about them. Realise that this is just a starting point.

TAP INTO YOUR SPIRIT GUIDE

Imagine you are walking along a path through a beautiful rainforest. Absorb all the sights, sounds and smells, enjoy the sensations of being in a rainforest. Keep walking until the path comes to a big field of purple flowers. Walk through the field and feel the flowers brush against your legs and the sunshine on your skin. Keep walking. In the distance, you see a beautiful temple with a staircase leading to the front door. Admire the temple's structure and shape. Notice how unique it is. Walk up the stairs and take notice of how the doors open magically on their own. Walk inside and look around until you meet your spirit guide. Your spirit guide may be anything—it may be an object, person, animal or just a voice or feeling. Ask your spirit guide what is great about you. Choose to be of service to yourself and choose to receive any image, object or words.

When you receive your image, slowly open your eyes and begin to write. Once you have described the message, think about it. What does it mean to you? Keep writing until you have written at least one page. Do not worry if you are making it all up as you go along, if you have chosen to be of service to yourself then the reading will be truthful. Don't think, just write.

How did you go? If you found this exercise difficult (or just weird), keep practising. You will learn to trust yourself and free up as you practise. If this written guidance is true, you will feel it in your body and your heart—your intuition will tell you it's true. It will seem to 'ring' true. If you are still not sure, try again.

Connecting with your dark side

See yourself sitting on a log by a dark, murky swamp. It is dark, cool and eerie.

Choose to be of service to yourself and receive any image, object or words that come to you. This is a symbol of the wound you created as a child when you did not receive complete validation of your parents' love. Once you have received the image, slowly open your eyes and write about what you have received, no matter how stupid or silly it may seem. From these thoughts, you can find out what you have been denying in your life.

Close your eyes again and choose to receive any image that represents what you have been denying in your life as a result of this wound. Once you have received a symbol, start writing. What does it mean to you?

DISCOVERING YOUR BELIEFS

Close your eyes again, choose to receive any image that represents the beliefs you created in relation to this wound. Once you have received a symbol, start writing. What does it mean to you?

WHAT STRATEGIES HAVE YOU DEVELOPED?

Close your eyes once more, choose to receive any image of the strategies you have created in relation to your beliefs. Once you have received a symbol, start writing. What does it mean to you?

THE REALITY YOU HAVE PERPETUATED

Close your eyes once more. Choose to receive any image of what you do to perpetuate the reality of hiding from this wound and your dark side. Once you have received a symbol, start writing. What does it mean to you?

STEPPING AWAY FROM YOUR WOUNDS

By embracing what you have been denying, you can create change.

Close your eyes once more and choose to receive any image of the step you need to take to embrace your dark side or wound. Once you have received a symbol, start writing. What does it mean to you?

SHARING YOUR GIFT

Close your eyes again. Choose to receive an image to show you what gift you have to help serve others. Once you have received a symbol, start writing. What does it mean to you?

EXERCISE EXAMPLE

I have a friend who has tried the above exercises and these are the thoughts that arose from working through them.

Wound
The image he received was a horrible monster. After considering it, he realised that his deep wound is that he thinks he is grotesque beyond imagination.

Denying
This friend is good looking and has an abundance of natural talents. He has been denying the truth of his physical beauty and his natural gifts.

Beliefs
He believes that he has to be mediocre, average and can't stand out. He believes he is not allowed to shine. He feels that if he embraces his beauty and natural gifts, he will be alone. He thinks he must entertain to get love.

Strategies
To prove that he is not grotesque, he is the consummate Mr Nice Guy. He is dismissive of compliments and acknowledgments. He has to prove how good he is to get people's approval.

Reality perpetuates
People only see a superficial person and don't take him seriously. People don't see that he has any substance as he believes people only want to know his superficial self. He convinces people that the veneer of himself is real.

Embracing what he denies
The image he received was a snake, where fierceness and killing is a part of life. There was no entertaining, no impressions to be made, he was just listening to the earth's vibrations, alert in the moment, as a snake would be. He wants to inspire people with his passion for making the most out of life.

His gift
To be of service, he needs to appreciate what he's got, rattle people's cages, make people aware that there is much to make of life. He needs to keep expressing his truth, through writing and music, with compassionate arrogance.

FINAL THOUGHTS ON THE REAL YOU

We have spent some time examining ourselves and you may feel uncomfortable discovering all the new things about yourself. Realising that you have been spending your whole life chasing goals to satisfy your egotistic beliefs and avoiding your dark side is confronting. Trying to achieve this transition overnight is impossible. It can take months to grasp the truth and accept your current reality and the strategies and beliefs you play out each day.

Live your life the way you truly want . . . your ego, your wounds and your beliefs will always be there, yet the choice about whether or not you live out these strategies is yours. Only you can engage your will to acknowledge what it is that you really want your life to be.

You need to discipline yourself by asking whether this is the life you really want and love, or do you want to keep living a façade? It can be a good idea to share your beliefs and strategies with your close friends so they can tell you if you are stuck in the mud or going for what you really want in life.

With perseverance you will discover all the qualities that make your life fulfilling. Remember:

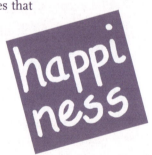

- You are already complete.
- You have beliefs and patterns that you engaged in to receive complete validation and love from your parents.
- Choose to be of service to yourself and others.
- Choose to do what you love in life.

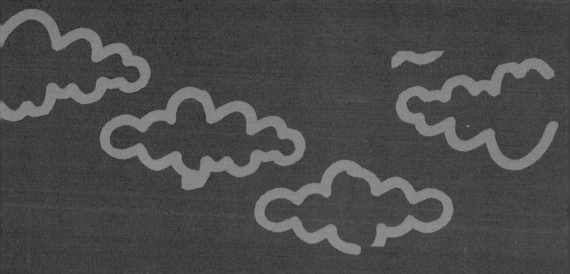

CHAPTER 9

CHOICES

Choices allow us to embrace our true self. We are free to choose what our real self wants. We create our life through our choices. Creating from choices is very different to goal setting. We make sure our choices are the things that we really want and not what our ego wants, which is often the case with goal setting. We then honestly look at the reality of what we have been doing to achieve this choice, and focus on the end result.

In his book, *The Path of Least Resistance*, Robert Fritz details the structure of creating what we want in our lives. I have adapted the structure from his teachings so that you can access these tools to create choices at will.

There are a few key premises as to how you can create what you really want in your life from choices.

PREMISES

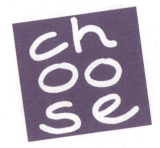

- You can create what you want in life
- Focus and belief creates your reality
- Tension seeks the fastest route to resolve itself
- Let intuition guide you
- Make it up
- Magic happens

YOU CAN CREATE WHAT YOU WANT IN LIFE

Sometimes we can feel like a fish stuck in a tank—trapped in our own world of limitations, fed by our ego, and limited by the boundaries of our beliefs and patterns. These things control, limit and define our lives.

You are creating everything that is happening in your life right now.

You do this consciously and unconsciously every moment of every day. Every decision you make will have an impact on your life. This is not necessarily a new idea, yet you could use this as a point of awakening for what you can do in your life.

People used to think the world was flat until other people started to prove it wasn't. Think about all those people who just seem to be able to do the impossible because they want to do it, despite what other people say and think. Sometimes trying something new involves trusting your intuition.

I make choices to get an end result. If I do not know what my end result is, then it is going to be hard to get it. This does not mean I have to have every detail of my life sorted out, it just means I need to have direction about what it is that I really want.

FOCUS AND BELIEF CREATE YOUR REALITY

Accepting that we can do what we want in our lives, all we need is focus and realisation to prevent us heading off course.

I remember when I was learning to hang-glide and I moved on to a course that was a little more difficult. As I took off, I was thrown off course. I turned and it seemed okay, but I did another turn and this time the wind took me further than I had anticipated. I headed straight to the bushes. My instructor said he saw my eyes looking at the bushes.

Where you look is where you will go.

Focus and belief create reality. This gem of information has pulled me through many a hairy situation while flying. I have learnt to focus on what I want and where I want to be, instead of where I don't want to be.

We have every right to choose what we want in our lives. Some people will never even think of choosing what they want to do in their lives because they have not embraced their real self (see Chapter 8). When you make a choice to do something, you take the power from what you don't want to do and put it into what you do want.

TENSION SEEKS THE FASTEST ROUTE TO RESOLVE ITSELF

Just as the water level in a dam begins to rise during a flood, tension builds as the water looks for a way to escape. It finds its escape route—a crack in the wall or over the top—and rushes with reckless abandon to its destination. The tension of an elastic band is similar. Pull on the elastic band and it will fling off, resolving the tension. Tension always tries to resolve itself.

For example, if you feel tension because you can't afford your ideal holiday, you could buy a guide book on the destination, book a flight to a more affordable destination, or set up a holiday bank account. If you manage to stay focused on what you want, rather than give in, you will become closer to achieving through choice.

Where you are is defined as your current reality. Where you want to be is your vision. Tension exists between your current reality and where you want to be.

LET INTUITION GUIDE YOU

Intuition is the ability to know when the right decision has been made. With intuition, you are guided by your truth rather than by your thoughts and feelings. It supersedes logic and often seems to work in weird and wonderful ways. Some people call it instinct, but, whatever you call it, when you know it's right, you know it's right.

I remember asking a friend, if she could do anything in her life, what would it be? One of her choices was to train at an international school in Canada. Another was to ride a horse through Mongolia. Then I asked her, if she went to that particular school what would she get out of it and where would it take her? She said she would be a skilled actor with acrobatic skills and that she would be more employable. I asked her, if she was more skilled, where would that take her? She said she would get a good acting job. All she really wanted to do was act! She had just finished an acting course so she could do this already!

This is an example of her beliefs and ego choosing what she did in her life. Her thoughts of not being good enough or perfect drove her to study more, to try and improve rather than act.

When I asked her what she would get from horseriding through Mongolia, it ended with the simple fact that she would be able to take in all the sights and sounds of Mongolia in a unique way. This was a true choice, because it didn't lead on to anything else in her life.

You need to distinguish between what 'the real you' wants and what your ego wants. The ego will always want to control you but it does not matter. You can deal with that by focusing on your choices of what you really want.

MAKE IT UP

Have you ever considered that we make up a lot of things in this world? Try the following exercise and see how many things, no matter how far you stretch them, are made up at one point in time.

A CHAIR IS A CHAIR . . . MAYBE

Look at what you are sitting on right now. Can you prove to me that what you are sitting on is real?

Here's an example of someone trying to prove it's real.

'I am sitting on the chair, I can feel it and see it.'

'How do you know that?'

'My nerves are sending signals from the surface of my skin, telling me it is making contact with an object. My eyes can see the shape and form of the chair which I am sitting on.'

'How do you know that?'

'From the knowledge I have gained over the years about how my brain, nervous system, eyes, and sense of touch works.'

'How do you know that?'

'I have read textbooks and seen documentaries where experts have told me this is how the body works.'

'How do you know that?'

'That is what research has shown.'

'How do you know that?'

'That is what I have read and seen.'

'How do you know that?'

'That is what I have remembered.'

'How do you know that?'

'I just have.'

'How do you know that?'

'I experience what I have remembered as images and ideas from past experiences.'

'How do you know that?'

'I feel it in my mind.'

'How do you know that?'

'I just do!'

'How do you know that?'

'I don't know how to explain it any more, I just do.'

'How do you know that?'

'I don't know, I guess I made it up.'

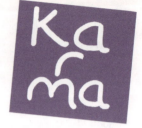

At some point in time, after working through the logic, we realise we have to make it up. The whole point of this exercise is to understand that even when we make something up, it can still be truthful. If you can understand how we make things up, you will be more open to making things up yourself, including what you need to validate your intuitive techniques.

When you use your intuition and have to interpret and make up what your symbols may mean, you can do it with conviction, realising it is worthwhile and real!

MAGIC HAPPENS

Just the other day a client agreed to teach me how to play the piano. The only problem was I didn't have a piano. I focused on getting a quality affordable piano. That same day, training a new client, I commented about the piano I saw in the house. The piano was for sale and within minutes I negotiated a contra deal. By the time I left, I had a beautiful piano. This is the magic of creation. Focus becomes reality. Focus on what you want, not what you don't want.

We call these sorts of events luck, synchronicity, karma and divine intervention. Making choices is just like that—deciding what you want to do, realising where you are at the present moment and then moving forward to get what you want.

Think about three things which you really wanted to create and how you managed to do them. Write down what you were focused on when you created them. Did you really want to create them? Did you believe that you could create them?

Magic happens!

When you decide you want something, you begin to experience tension. Perhaps you have chosen to go on a trek in the Himalayas. Pretty soon you will start doubting yourself, worrying about how much it will cost, how difficult it will be, what you need to learn about climbing. Before you know it, the tension has increased so much that the whole idea of going to the Himalayas is just too hard.

If you are unable to sit with this tension and focus on what you want, you will cave into the pressure and look to resolve the tension by cancelling the trip or changing the destination to somewhere easier.

BASIC INTUITION EXERCISE

To help you find what you want to do in life, you use a few main principles. First, you establish the vision, then you need to be aware of your current reality so that you can create some structural tension to help you head towards your vision. Then you need to find out your next step. The easiest way to do this is to use your intuition.

Using your intuition may be confronting if you have never tried it before, however, the more you do it, the better you will get. Try to keep an open mind and see what you come up with.

1. Make sure you are comfortable and close your eyes. Take in a big breath and let out a big sigh, 'Aaaaaaarrrrgggghhhh'. Now take in another big breath and let that go with a sigh as well.
2. Acknowledge (mentally) any thoughts and feelings you might have at this present time. It does not matter what they are, this is just a starting point. This exercise makes contact your gut instinct by interpreting any symbols or objects that arise in your mind.

3. Choose to be of service to yourself (or to the other person if you are helping someone else). Take a big breath and allow the breath to completely go.

4. Imagine yourself transforming into a beautiful white mist. Feel your whole body release. Feel how soft and cool you have become.

5. Imagine a tunnel. Allow yourself to be drawn into the tunnel. Feel yourself as a mist being sucked upwards, going faster and faster. Feel yourself becoming brighter and brighter as you travel faster and faster up the tunnel.

6. At the end of this tunnel, you arrive at a wonderful place where everything you ever wished for is there. This is your land of plenty. Make a conscious decision to find your particular vision if you already have one in mind and notice all the wonderful qualities about it. Enjoy it, know that you can create it.

7. Choose to receive any image, word or thought that comes to you. When you feel you have come up with something, slowly open your eyes and start to write. Keep writing and don't stop until you've written at least one page. Make it up if you have to. As long as you have chosen to be of service to yourself, then what you write will be true.

You have just established your vision. You now need to establish some structural tension to help you move towards your vision.

Sometimes the choices we make aren't our real choices. To ensure they are real choices, not from the ego, ask yourself, 'If I get this, what will I have?' For example, if I said I wanted a black Porsche, I would ask, 'What would I have if I get this car?'

I could cruise the streets, and impress the girls.

If I could cruise the streets and impress the girls, what would that give me?

I might be able to pick up.

What would that give me?

I might be able to sleep with a beautiful person.

What would that give me?

Just that, being able to sleep with that person.

The real choice in this situation, as crass as it may seem, is to sleep with a beautiful person, not drive the car. However, if I chose to have a black Porsche to drive a beautiful sports car and enjoy the superb performance and handling, then that would be a real choice.

RECEIVING YOUR CREATIONS

It is important to acknowledge what you have created in your life. Write down what you have already created in the past couple of years that have been really important to you.

- What have you learnt from these creations?
- What have you changed and now do differently?
- Acknowledge and honour what has been both great and petty in your life recently, and then ask what is the most important thing to let go of?

If you have lots of choices, sometimes you can get confused about what you should focus on. You can use your intuition to find out which will be the best to focus on. The more you actively use your intuition, the faster you will become at creating choices. I work through a choice every day. I do an intuition exercise on the vision, current reality and next step.

Remember you can always keep yourself focused by asking yourself, 'What do I want?' This helps to keep you on track.

PROBLEM SOLVING

Rather than rationally coming up with solutions to problems, our intuition can often come up with a next-step solution free from our ego's interference. To make sure that you have given your rational mind a chance, write down a few rational solutions to a problem you have.

Now let's use your intuition.

Use the same intuition exercise as before, but this time substitute your vision with what you would love to get out of the situation or problem. Write down what you receive and make it up.

Be aware that sometimes your action may not address the problem in the way you expected, but it will take you towards what you really want. It is worth noting that often we spend a lot of our time trying to resolve problems rather than just doing what we want. When we go for what we love, the problems tend to disappear. Are you trying to avoid doing what you really want by resolving problems?

PROBLEM-SOLVING EXERCISE

Think of a problem you have. As an example, some time ago I couldn't get my housemate to pay his phone bills on time. The rational solutions were to boot him out of house or to keep hassling him for money.

Now let's try intuition with this problem.

Make sure you are comfortable and close your eyes. Take in a big breath and let out a big sigh, 'Aaaaaaarrrrgggghhhh'. Acknowledge (mentally) any thoughts and feelings you might have, it does not matter what they are.

Imagine yourself walking through a beautiful forest. Imagine the details of your special forest—the leaves on the trees, the plants, the birds, the smell, the aroma, the path you are walking on, the sounds of the birds, animals, insects, your foot steps. Keep walking for a minute or so.

Come out into a field full of purple flowers. Walk through the field, enjoying the colours of the flowers and the smells and textures. In the middle of the field is a beautiful temple—your temple, a shrine for you alone. Head towards this temple and the steps and the doors. As you climb the steps, the doors open magically for you and you walk inside.

Look around inside the temple and enjoy what you see. Notice that in the middle of this temple is a small cot. When you look inside this cot, you see a baby. This baby is you. Notice how innocent, calm, complete and natural you are.

Now allow yourself to feel what it is like to be this baby—innocent, wide-eyed, safe and complete. Enjoy this sensation of innocence and make a conscious decision to be of service to your higher self. Ask yourself, 'What is the highest truth to the problem I am are facing?' Choose to receive any image, word or thought that comes to you. When you feel you have come up with something, open your eyes.

Write it down and make it up.

For my problem I came up with an image of giving my housemate a sword. This way I could empower him to take responsibility. I followed this up by telling my housemate about his responsibilities. He soon paid all his bills, and he got another phone line connected so he could take responsibility for his own phone costs.

We can get stuck trying to resolve our problems rationally, yet, when we use our intuition, we often take it one step further—resolving the problem and getting closer to what we want in our lives.

Remember, focus creates reality! Become aware of how easy it is to use a rational approach to solving things, yet how quickly we can find a solution using our intuition.

CHAPTER 10

EXPRESSION

The need to express yourself, your emotions, thoughts and feelings is very important. The fun part is learning new ways to express yourself and communicate. I have included a list of fun activities that can help to foster avenues of expression. Some may seem a little odd and others may be just what you need. Remember that life is not one-size-fits-all. What works for you may not work for others. We all have different learning preferences—visual, auditory, or kinaesthetic. If you know which learning preferences you have, it may indicate why you have the burning desire to take up painting, writing, singing or dancing.

Writing exercises

These exercises will improve your ability to express yourself through words.

Sunrise notes

Put some paper and a pen beside your bed at night so you can start writing first thing in the morning.

Write three pages. Don't stop until you have finished all three pages. Keep writing even if you write, 'I don't know what to write about'. The exercise is all about getting it out onto paper.

You may feel you are sacrificing some precious morning time but you will improve your communication skills and unlock some of the issues that are going on in your life. Quite often, simple solutions begin to appear as well as inspirational ideas.

Journal

Journals are about communicating our thoughts, feelings and emotions. We can capture inspirational ideas, find clarity and even laugh at what is happening in our lives. Find an inspirational book, one with an appealing cover, in which to write. You may be further inspired by a pen kept aside especially for your journal thoughts.

You can write in your journal anytime, but the more often you write the more you will gain.

VERBAL EXPRESSION

Speak and thou shall be heard! Many of us fall into the trap of letting things slip by, because we fail to speak up. Keeping quiet kills our confidence and our ability to communicate and express ourselves. No matter how stupid or insignificant your ideas may seem, it is better to bring them out into the open rather than allow them to fester inside, unheard.

I used to think more than what I let come out of my mouth. What was going on in my mind was perfectly clear to me, but I was not communicating. Unfortunately, this led to the end of a long-term relationship. It did, however, bring home the realisation that my communication skills were so poor.

FOREIGN LANGUAGE EXPERIENCE

Imagine you are in a foreign country, with no understanding of the language. You are lost in a town and are hungry and want to find something to eat, a train or bus to get you to a hotel, or somewhere to sleep. You have to make up your own ways to communicate what you want.

Use your imagination. Use your voice, body or drawings to communicate what you want.

and then.....
I was disco
dancing in
this amazing
room with a
dazzling disco
ball, pulling
these wild moves
.... and then...

VISUAL COMMUNICATION

DRAWING

Many of you may have heard of the concept of drawing from the right side of the brain. Basically, when you draw things, you use the left side of your brain, the side controlled by rational and logical thoughts. You tend to draw one thing at a time, and what you draw looks a particular way. Unfortunately, this disrupts the flow so much that the drawings usually look decidedly unlike what we really wanted to draw.

When you use the right side of the brain, you tend to use your intuitive perception, see things as a whole, and provide a more realistic representation of what you see. The right side of the brain is something that needn't be relegated to just the visual arts.

Most of us have been trained to engage the left side of the brain when we process information, using linear approaches to solve problems. When we engage the right side, we start to become intuitive and see problems as a whole, processing information while simultaneously using mental images freely. So let's start.

Using your opposite hand to the one you normally use, pick up a fat marker, crayon or texta. Try not to use any fine-detail tool like a pen or technical pencil, we want fat lines. Draw the house you grew up in. It does not matter what you think it should look like, just draw anything that you think conveys the image. Try not to think too much about it, just remember what it used to look like. Don't look at the paper while drawing, just draw. Do not correct your drawing, leave it as it is. And don't criticise yourself.

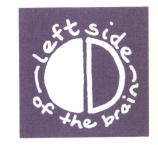

INTUITIVE SCULPTURE EXERCISE

Collect five objects from outside and combine them to create an inspirational piece. Try not to think about it too much, just let it happen. You'll be surprised by your result if you create using your intuition only.

USING NEGATIVE SPACE

When drawing or painting, becoming aware of the negative space around an object can help you to engage the right side of your brain. What you choose to focus on can affect your skills. If you can look at the spaces around and in between objects, you can use these to construct a drawing without thinking about what the object must look like, and you'll end up with a much fresher representation of what's in front of you.

A classic example is when you have two faces opposite each other. You can see the image in a number of ways, either as one object in the middle or two faces looking at each other.

Try placing three bottles or simple objects in front of you. Make sure they are all slightly apart so that you can see space between each object. Now grab a black marker or crayon and, with your normal writing hand, start filling in the spaces between the shapes and around them—don't draw the acutal bottles or objects. Don't worry about what the shapes you are drawing are, just focus on the spaces in between and around the objects. Keep looking at the scene in front of you as much as possible. When you are finished, step back and admire the end result—note how strong the drawing is.

Try not to criticise what you have done. It is just a start to expressing yourself. We don't all have to take up drawing and become famous artists. Rather, it is a great way to engage the right side of the brain. Through this can start to develop the ability to communicate some of your ideas visually. Whether it's a presentation or report needed at work, or ways you can arrange your furniture in the living room, drawing is a way of expressing yourself. You'll find that as you draw the subconscious affects your pencil strokes or paintbrush techniques and you are left with a little piece of yourself transposed onto your art piece.

You can express yourself further through sculpture, painting, drawing or photography.

AUDITORY COMMUNICATION

Have you ever noticed how your voice expresses your emotions? A clear, well-projected voice helps us to articulate what we want to communicate.

Our vocal chords are mini muscles, and we need to develop them if we want to increase their capabilities. The voice is one of our most beautiful gifts. Every voice is unique. The articulation of words, tone of the voice, volume and resonance are all things which make us sound the way we do.

I notice that when my confidence wanes, my voice becomes softer, I start to speak through the corner of my mouth and I speak in a nasally voice. It hampers my ability to really express myself. The exercises below will help you to gain confidence in yourself and your voice.

Laughing exercise

Put your fingers around your throat lightly and start speaking. Feel what happens with your vocal chords. Now laugh and feel it in your throat. Notice how it expands and opens the airway? This is what we want when speaking or singing—it allows an uninhibited voice to come through.

If you feel nervous before an important meeting, you can use this exercise to make your voice stronger and feel more confident. Laugh loudly and confidently.

Tongue twister exercises

To sharpen the tongue and lip coordination, say some of the following quickly:

Granny's golden goose greedily gobbles golden grain.
Six sleek swans swam swiftly southwards.
Green glass globes glow greenly.
I wish to wash my Irish wristwatch.
She said she should sit!
Peter Piper picked a peck of pickled peppers.
A peck of pickled peppers Peter Piper picked.
If Peter Piper picked a peck of pickled peppers, where's the peck of pickled peppers Peter Piper picked?
A big black bug bit a big black bear, made the big black bear bleed blood.
I slit the sheet, the sheet I slit, and on the slitted sheet I sit.
She sells seashells by the seashore.

The shells she sells are surely seashells.

So if she sells shells on the seashore, I'm sure she sells seashore shells.

I am not the pheasant plucker, I'm the pheasant plucker's mate. I am only plucking pheasants 'cause the pheasant plucker's running late.

How much wood would a woodchuck chuck if a woodchuck could chuck wood? He would chuck, he would, as much as he could, and chuck as much wood as a woodchuck would if a woodchuck could chuck wood.

After trying these for a while, you soon begin to realise how slack you can be when a r t i c u l a t i n g words.

NASAL EXERCISES

If you can develop a distinction between nasal and non-nasal sounds, your voice can become a more powerful, wide-ranging tool to use when expressing yourself. Try making the sound that kids use to tease others in the school playground— neah, neah, neah, neah, neah . . .

Try singing the vowel 'a', as in 'AAAAARRRRRRR'. Don't worry about how it sounds. First sing it softly, then loudly, then back to soft again. Then try singing the note going from loud to soft then back to loud all in one breath.

When we become nervous, the voice tends to be quieter and people have trouble hearing us. Pull back your shoulders, lift up your chin and fire away! 'AAAARRRRRRRRR . . .'

STOPPING AND STARTING, INTONATION, EMPHASIS

Listen to a news presenter and notice the intonation and emphasis of their voice. If we all speak at one pitch and rhythm, our voices are boring. Notice how at the end of a serious story a news presenter will end a sentence with a lower pitch. Yet when there is an uplifting story the voice will have a higher pitch.

Read the following passage and emphasise the important words. Try to increase the volume when you see this symbol +++ and decrease when you see ——. Try to raise the pitch of your voice when you see ∧∧∧ and lower the pitch down when you see ∨∨∨.

The door swung open and Christopher and John ran down the hallway. They stood before him, breathless and smiling. —— They had her eyes. His grip softened, —— his heart dropped to the pit of his stomach, +++ but then ∧∧∧ somehow his heart grew wings and started to fly. He flew back to the +++ time when he looked into her eyes and was —— immersed in her love. He still loved her. They were the proof of it. ∨∨∨ The knife dropped to the floor.

Christopher stared at him, eyes wide and gasped, +++ 'Dad, what are you doing?'

Practising this passage with the intonations will give your voice more animation and most importantly people will enjoy the words you express and communicate to them.

FALLING BOMB (SOUND UP AND DOWN IN PITCH)

This exercise increases the range of voice from high to low. The more musical your voice is in terms of pitch, the more interesting it is to listen to.

Start with a high-pitched sound and slowly lower the pitch like the sound of a bomb falling from the sky. When you reach the bottom of your range, come back up to the original high pitch as smoothly as possible.

MOVEMENT AND GESTURE EXERCISES

You can have fun with your body when expressing yourself. I have an Italian friend who is always teaching me a few Italian phrases, which I comically repeat with as much fervour, excitement and passion as I think deserved of the Italian culture. This includes amazingly exaggerated whirring hands and arms flying around the place as I say to passersby 'Bvipuvbnvwinvnweoivmerte sula musica'. (No I do not like tennis. Please put on some music.) Some cultures use their body more than others.

Why not try adding a little more body movement into your life for a bit more excitement and passion, you could even touch!

TOUCHING

Some people may touch you more when they talk to you than others. Not necessarily because they like you, but because they are kinaesthetic and they express themselves through touch. Try touching to communicate and see if it works for you. Touch someone in a particular way—stroke their hair, give them a big hug, hold a hand. Be careful not to offend the other person. Some people don't like to be touched—more's the pity as it's a beautiful way to connect.

DANCING

Dancing is a great way of expressing yourself—even if you don't have 'the moves' you'd like. Put on some of your favourite music. Wear a blindfold and move to the music.

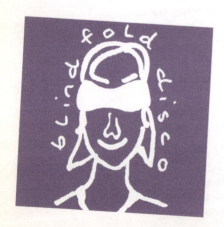

How do you feel? Angry, happy, sad, tired, pepped up? Just allow your free flowing movement to reflect how you are feeling. If you're angry, maybe you want to stomp your feet. If you are tired, you might want to drag your feet. If you are revved up, you may want to spin or jump. Just let yourself do whatever you feel inclined to do. Use your arms, your head, your hands, your feet, your fingers and toes, your face, your lips and tongue, everything—go for it. Enjoy! Dance for as long as you want, have no limitations. When you are finished, take off your blindfold, turn off the music and write down how you feel.

Staring into each other's eyes

Find a partner, preferably someone you don't know, or even better someone you don't get on with particularly well. Sit opposite them and look in their eyes. It will feel uncomfortable at first and you will want to look away and close your eyes. All kinds of things will come up for you but try to avoid looking away. If you are finding it really hard, take in a huge breath and let out a big sigh.

I always find this difficult, but I realise how much it reveals. Stick with it, you may even start to laugh. Does your partner have a dominant eye? What colour are their eyes? What else can you see in there? Keep looking at their eyes for at least five minutes.

When you have finished, discuss what occurred for each of you. What emotions came up? Were you intimidated, nervous, confident?

We use our eyes every day to convey messages to people, either intentionally or unintentionally. They reveal a lot. Next time you meet someone, try to look into their eyes and see what is revealed to you. See what you can learn and become aware of how the connection between you has changed because of it.

A walk in life

Think about how you walk down the street. Do you run, do you look down at the pavement, or check yourself out in the shop window? Do you acknowledge people passing by or are you strutting like a model on a catwalk?

It is suggested that the speed people walk reflects their level of confidence and direction in life. Sometimes I subscribe to this idea, however, walking with purpose and awareness is a quality which many 'quick' walkers never choose to experience because they are not concerned about expression and the joys of body movement, nor are they aware of what is going on around them.

Why not feel the difference yourself. Try a power walk, followed by a strutting sexual walk. Then try a meditative walk, experiencing every footstep and movement in the body. Experiment with where you are looking and what you are taking in on your journey. Have fun with it.

Power walk

In your power walk, try to look and feel super powerful. Swing the elbows, engage the upper body, lift your head, feel the breeze on your face, pull your shoulders back and take big powerful strides. Enjoy the planting of the feet as you walk along.

Strutting sexual walk

Imagine you are walking on a line. Place every step down the centre of that line. Be loose in your upper body and allow your arms to swing naturally. Breathe into the belly and let go of the hips. Keep your chin and head lifted.

Meditative walk

You can do this at any pace, but it does tend to work best when you have a bit of time, with few distractions. The principle is to walk with awareness.

Focus on one thing only. Start by finding somewhere ahead of you for the eyes to rest on. A nice tree or building. You don't need to look at the ground as much as you think when you walk. Your peripheral vision will take care of you. Just feel yourself being drawn to the object.

Become aware of the sensation in your right foot, and work through the body methodically—right big toe, second toe, third toe etc. Work up the right leg and hips, then move onto the abdominal area, chest, back and shoulders. Then become aware of your left foot and work up as before. Move onto your right hand, arm etc. If the mind wanders, bring it back and refocus. Enjoy the sensation of the walking movement in the body.

Focus on the rolling of the foot, the bending of the knee, the flexing of the calf and thigh, the swing of the hips and arms, the position of the head. Feel how the breath comes in and out. See how the body changes with each step.

Can you breathe more freely, and reduce tension and control? Ponder on what comes naturally and how much you can control your body movement, even when you might think you are just walking! Just let go and enjoy.

Use your imagination in this exercise to put intention behind the action. Walk slowly in an open space. Imagine you are walking along the beach in the evening. Enjoy the casual feelings that come to mind.

Now walk a bit faster, as if you are rushing to the shops to get something.

Then a bit faster to get to the bus stop.

Now go really fast to make sure you get to the bus on time.

Then imagine you're busting to go to the toilet and walk even faster.

Now start to work back through the different images, coming back down to the slowest stage—walking on the beach.

Now just walk and feel the rhythm of your body. Feel how the foot is grounded—are your feet turned in or out? Don't change it, just feel it. Work up the calves, thighs, hips, arms, chest. Are your thumbs in or out? Be aware of all the joints in your body and how they are moving. Does one arm move further than the other? Swing your hips, and your arms. Drop your shoulders, stick your bum out and have a giggle at yourself and feel what your body is experiencing.

Honesty hour

An amazing friend taught me this great exercise. If you have a partner or a really close friend, this is a great opportunity to talk about what's going on in each other's lives.

Go somewhere where both of you feel very comfortable. Being honest and speaking the truth is the only stipulation. If you feel you can't look the person in the eyes, lay down, close your eyes and talk about anything that is going on in your life.

When you are listening, be attentive. Think how hard it must be for the other person to reveal themselves to you. Speak your truth as well and share this wonderful opportunity to bare your soul.

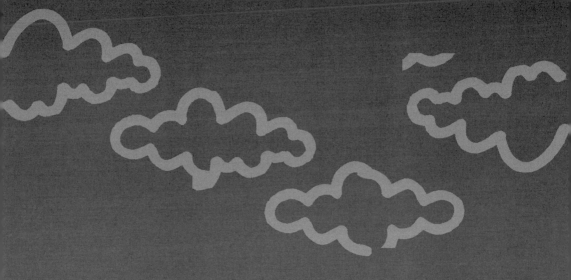

CONCLUSION

By now, I hope that you have realised the importance of looking after your life and how to make the most of it. The journey does not end there. For many of us, it may just be beginning, for others it is the continuation of a path we have been travelling for some time.

If this book has made a difference to you, then the rewards that will come from stepping into your life are boundless.

Life's Little Toolbox is a guide that I use constantly in my own life—for the times I feel down, stressed, not communicative or just uncreative. It gives me the quick tools to help me do what I really want to do.

Behind each page there are a thousand more. The art of Zen is to make more with less. I hope I have achieved this in this book. This is by no means the be-all and end-all of books for wellbeing—if it inspires you to read and practice more in this area, fantastic, and, if it's just enough for you, I am equally stoked.

I look forward to your readership as you embark on your journey and continue to use *Life's Little Toolbox* when necessary.

Big smile,

Nils

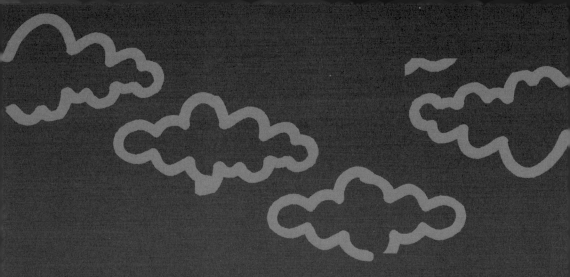

RECOMMENDED READING AND RESOURCES

The Alchemist: A fable about following your dream, by Paulo Coelho, Harper Perennial
  edition, New York, 1998.
The Art of Happiness: A handbook for Living, by His holiness the Dalai Lama and Howard
  C. Cutler, MD, Hodder Headline, Sydney, 1998.
The Art of War, by Sun Tzu, translated by Thomas Cleary, Shambhala Pocket Classics,
  Boston, 1991.
The Celestine Prophecy: An adventure, by James Redfield, Bantam Books, USA, 1994.
Change Your Thinking, by Dr Sarah Edelman, ABC Books, Sydney, 2002.
The Complete Book of Abs, by Kurt Brungardt, Villard Books, New York, 1994.
Creative Wisdom for Writers, by Roland Fishman, Allen & Unwin, Sydney, 2000.
*Drawing on the Right Side of the Brain: A course in enhancing creativity and artistic
  confidence*, by Betty Edwards, J. P. Tarcher, Los Angeles, 1979.
Do it Now: Break the procrastination habit, by William J. Knaus, John Wiley & Sons, 1998.
The Enneagram: Understanding yourself and the others in your life, by Helen Palmer
  HarperCollins, San Francisco, 1991.
Glucose Revolution: The groundbreaking medical discovery of the GI factor, by Dr Anthony
  Leeds, Assoc. Prof. Jenny Brand Miller, Kaye Foster Powell and Dr Stephen
  Golaguri, Hodder & Stoughton, 2001.
The Heart of Yoga, by T.K.V Desikachar, Inner Traditions International, Vermont, 1995.
How Meditation Heals the Body and Mind, by Eric Harrison, Perth Meditation Centre,
  Perth, 1999.
If Not Dieting, Then What?, by Dr Rick Kausman, Allen & Unwin, Sydney, 1998.
Johnathon Livingston Seagull: A story, by Richard Bach, Avon Books, New York, 1970.
The Kybalion: A study of the Hermetic philosophy of Ancient Egypt and Greece, by Three
  Initiates, The Yogi Publication Society, Masonic Temple, Chicago ILL, 1940.
Manhood: An action plan for changing men's lives, by Steve Biddulph, Finch, Sydney,
  1995.
*Men Are from Mars, Women Are from Venus: A practical guide for improving communi-
  cation and getting what you want in your relationships*, by John Gray, HarperCollins,
  New York, 1993.
The New Golf Paradigm, by Kris Barkway with Tunku Halimm, Pelanduk Publications,
  Malaysia, 2001.

The Okinawa Way: How to improve your health and longevity dramatically, by J. Willcox, MD, D. Craig Willcox, PhD, and Makoto Suzuki, MD, Penguin Books, London, 2001.

The Path of Least Resistance: Learning to become the creative force in your own life, by Robert Fritz, Fawcett Columbine, New York, 1989.

The Seven Spiritual Laws of Success: A practical guide to the fulfillment of your dreams, by Deepak Chopra, Bantam Press, London, 1996.

Sexual Secrets for Men, by Kerry Riley, Random House, Sydney, 2001.

Strong Women Stay Slim, by Miriam E. Nelson PhD with Sarah Wernwick PhD, Bantam Doubleday Dell Pub, 1999.

Taoist Secrets of Love, by Mantak Chia, Aura Press, New York, 1994.

Teach Yourself to Meditate (second edition), by Eric Harrison, Simon & Schuster, Sydney, 1998.

Thought for the Today: Positive Thinking Series 1, Brahma Kumaris World Spiritual University, Raja Yoga Mediation, 1988 BK Media Resource International, Sydney.

Wake Up Your Creative Genius, by Kurt Hanks and Jay Parry, Crisp Publications, California, 1991.

When I Loved Myself Enough, by Kim McMillen with Alison McMillen, Pan Macmillan, Sydney, 2001.

Useful links

Mental Health
www.depression.net
www.mentalhelp.net/psyhelp
www.stress.org

Health improvement programs
Active for Life: www.active.org.uk
Fitsmart.com
Okinawa way: www.okinawaway.com

Health resources

Australian Department of Health and Aged care. www.health.gov.au
MayoClinic.com: www.mayohealth.org
Ministry of Health (NZ): www.moh.govt.nz
Reality Check: www.realitycheck.org.au

American Diabetes Association: www.diabetes.org
Diabetes Australia: www.dav.org.au
International Diabetes Federation: www.idf.org
Juvenile Diabetes Foundation: www.jdrf.org
Multilingual diabetes site: www.multilingualdiabetes.org

American Cancer Society: www.cancer.org
Australian Cancer Society: www.cancer.org.au
Cancer Help (UK): www.cancerhelp.org.uk
Cancer Society of New Zealand: www.cancernz.org.nz

Arthritis Foundation: www.arthritis.org
National Osteoporosis Society: www.nos.org.uk
National Osteoporosis Foundation: www.nof.org

American Heart Association: www.americanheart.org
American Stroke Foundation: www.strokeassociation.org
Heart Foundation of Australia: www.heartfoundation.com.au
Heart Foundation of New Zealand: www.nhf.org.nz
National Stroke Foundation: www.alznsw.asn.au
The Stroke Foundation: www.stroke.org.uk

Nutrition

American Obesity Association: www.obesity.org
American Dietetic Association: www.eatright.org
Australian New Zealand Food Authority: www.anzfa.gov.au
Automatic Body Mass Index Calculation: www.bodymassindex.com
British Nutrition Foundation: www.nutrition.org.uk

Canadian Dieticians: www.dieticians.ca
Vegetarian Resource Group: www.vrg.org

Personal Development
www.livingfromgreatness.com.au
www.mindtools.com
www.tantragoddesoz.com

Other
National Self-help Clearinghouse: www.selfhelpweb.org
Look for a Book: www.lookforabook.com

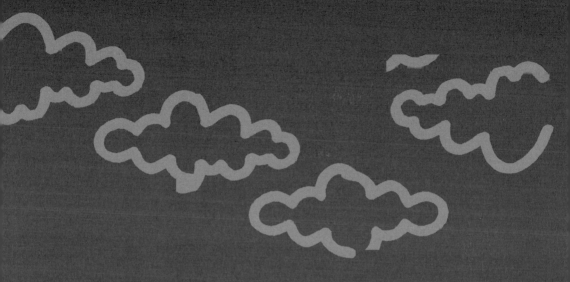

ACKNOWLEDGMENTS

To my parents for bringing me into this world, their wisdom, travelling, love of the country, and their unerring support despite the wayward path I have taken through the years. Thank you, I love you heaps!

To Kris McIntyre, for all her love and help in the early editing, her tireless support and words of encouragement.

To Bill Tikos, my esteemed agent, whose guidance and enthusiasm helped me to complete the project, and whose valuable skills ensured its publication.

To my commissioning editor, Jo Paul, for having faith in the project and fearlessly testing the exercises in her office in clear view of her team. And also for her kind words telling me what to chop away to reveal the masterpiece beneath. To my editor, Alexandra Nahlous, for her attention to detail and all the ways we could package the book.

To my fantastic designer, the intrepid Louise Davis from Mathematics, for her design skills and thoughtful regard for my simple drawings. I still owe you a thousand shiatsus!

To Louise Remond, Clinical Psychologist Royal North Shore Hospital and the University of Technology, for all her wisdom and love over the years, her constructive criticism on the healthy mind and for forgiving all the mistakes I have made.

To Caitlin Ekerick, for her encouragement, and first reading of a completely confusing manuscript, which only resulted in positive feedback.

To Janet Franklin, esteemed dietician at Royal Prince Alfred Hospital, who taught me so much about nutrition, and for having the modesty to allow someone with such inferior knowledge to explain it to the readers.

To Lorraine Rushton, who helped me with the yoga classes, whose teaching inspired me to become a yoga teacher, and whose constant support ensured I had classes to teach and learn from. Big hug!

To Emma, the amazing acupuncturist/yoga teacher/school teacher. Thank you for working on my leg to help me run again and for introducing me to the intricacies of acupuncture and helping me with the pressure points.

To Darren Ward, from Living from Greatness, for his intuitive genius and encouragement, advice and friendship, and the encouragement to write what I believed in and to articulate my philosophy on life, which has become this book. Lots of love.

To all my teachers and students, who have taught me so much.

To my big brother and his family, whom I may have neglected whilst committing myself to this project, for their support and early encouragement in expression.

To Kris Barkway, for his intuitive skills and prowess in teaching me golf and how my game reflects my life.

To Paul Moss for his great yoga photography.

To all my friends, for our friendships and relationships that bring so much love, fun and meaning to my life.

Thank you.

Nils